ECHOES
——— FROM THE ———
OPERATING ROOM
Vignettes in Surgical History

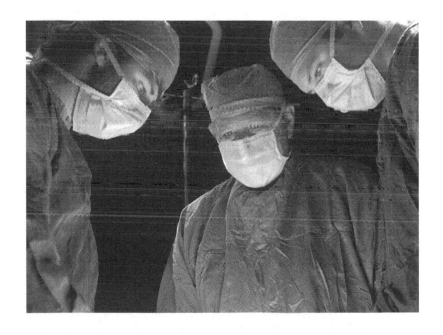

Carl R. Boyd, MD

Order this book online at www.trafford.com
or email orders@trafford.com

Most Trafford titles are also available at major online book retailers.

Cover photograph operative scene from Provident Hospital
(Circa 1930): Lee Russell photographer, Collection of the Library of Congress
(public domain) and original photography and editing by B. Davidson 2012.

Title page photograph: by K. Roeder. Subjects: M. Gage Ochsner Jr.,
M.D. FACS, M. Gage Ochsner III, and Matthew Cousins Ochsner

Printed in the United States of America.

ISBN: 978-1-4669-7753-2 (sc)
ISBN: 978-1-4669-7755-6 (hc)
ISBN: 978-1-4669-7754-9 (e)

Library of Congress Control Number: 2013901173

Trafford rev. 01/21/2013

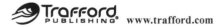 www.trafford.com

North America & international
toll-free: 1 888 232 4444 (USA & Canada)
phone: 250 383 6864 ♦ fax: 812 355 4082

This book is dedicated to Mims Gage Ochsner, Jr., M.D., esteemed teacher, respected colleague, and master surgeon. His influence will echo in our hearts and minds for years to come.

CONTENTS

Addendum: Presidential Patients

1

A Moment in Montgomery

I think I should begin by telling you, the reader, a little about my own surgical history and why I wrote this book. I was twenty years old when I walked into my first operating room at St. Margaret's Hospital in Montgomery, Alabama. After graduating from high school, I lived at home in Louisville, Kentucky in order to attend the University of Louisville. But after eighteen months of very little study, my two major interests were rock and roll and Kentucky bourbon. At the end of a late night of too much of both, the Beatles blared out from the radio in my 1957 Chevy, cutting through my aimless adolescent confusion, and told me with their song's title that I was a "Nowhere Man". This unlikely instance of clarity suddenly took my life in a different direction. That same morning I joined the United States Air Force in order to grow up and to help my country, or so I thought, in Viet Nam. It was 1966 and the war was escalating rapidly to its peak. The recruiter assigned me to be a medic. After basic training, and then medic school, I was told I was to be an operating room technician. I was stationed in Montgomery, Alabama for training. After a week of learning the names of the instruments, the correct way to fold linens, and the details of sterile technique, Master Sergeant Cartledge sent me downtown to St. Margaret's to watch surgery for the first time.

The head nurse, who was a tall imposing Catholic nun, told me to go to room two, stay out of the way, and just watch. Doing as I was told, I found operating room two and pushed open the two half doors that hung in mid-air from each side frame much like the old bar room doors in a Roy Rogers western movie. The moment I stepped into that small operating room in Montgomery, Alabama, my life was changed forever. The surgeon was making an incision into a young man's knee. I knew at that second what I would do for the rest of my life. I had never seen anything so exciting, so interesting, so precise, and so meaningful. I knew I had to do it. That moment in Montgomery hit me like a thunderbolt from Zeus. I hurried back to my sergeant to tell him that I finally knew what I wanted to do, so he could let me go back to the University of Louisville and I could become a surgeon. Upon hearing this, after his laughter had stopped, he assured me that I had four more years to serve in "this man's Air Force" and that if I lived through Viet Nam then I could try college again.

I spent three more years in Air Force operating rooms with one of those years being stationed in Southeast Asia at U-Tapoa Air Force Base in Thailand. The horrible injuries and wounds I saw there did not deter me but further reinforced my desire to be the one making the decisions and doing the dissection. When I came home and was discharged, I immediately returned to the University of Louisville and started college all over again. I had but one goal and that was to become a surgeon, not a doctor, but a surgeon. After graduating college, the University of Kentucky accepted me into medical school and gave me the chance to get a M.D. degree. Then five years of intense training in surgical residency followed, and now some 30 years as an attending professor of surgery has passed since that fateful day in my first operating room. I have had the privilege of operating on many thousands of patients and the opportunity to teach hundreds of young men and women the satisfaction of caring for patients in and out of the operating room.

When I returned home and reentered college, I worked as a scrub technician for a truly talented surgeon named Benjamin B. Jackson. He had trained under the great professor of surgery Robert Ritchie Linton at Harvard and the Massachusetts General

Hospital. Every day, as we operated, Dr. Jackson recounted the Greek myths and told story after story about the great surgeons of the past. I was always quizzed the next day on the details of that day's history lesson. He instilled in me a love for both Greek mythology and surgical history. He was my first surgeon mentor and had a great impact on me. My son bears his name and, in a way, he is partly responsible for this book.

This book is dedicated to the ones that came before and is for those who will come after. It is written for those young men and women who have allowed me to teach them and in return have taught me even more. The appreciation of the history of surgery is not just for old surgeons. It adds a foundation, understanding, and a certain grace to the practice of all of those involved in a profession that is itself ageless.

Every day in every operating room throughout the world the same names are spoken over and over again. These names are the names of the great surgical innovators and teachers of the past. These men have become eponyms. Surgeons call out for Kocher clamps and Deaver retractors. They perform Billroth gastric resections and Bassini hernia repairs. Those names and all the others have echoed from the bright clean environment of operating rooms for over a hundred years. This little work attempts to tell their stories in an educational and entertaining way while at the same time honoring those names and their contributions that formed the basis of modern day surgery.

As the years pass by, I increasingly think of the skill and courage of those that came before me. I know that they too must have felt the weight and loneliness of life and death decisions. I know that they too experienced the quiet and inward exhilaration of the operative procedure completed perfectly just as planned and without complication. But I can only imagine the courage and brilliance it took to take that next innovative step into the unknown and do it with the patient's life in the balance.

Even today as I finish scrubbing my hands, when I back through that operating room door and step into the sanctum of surgery, I can hear those echoes of the past and feel their presence. Even now at the close of my career, it is still the same excitement for me and still the same thunderbolt as it was that moment in Montgomery.

A Short History of Medicine

2000 B.C.—"Here, eat this root."
1000 B.C.—"That root is heathen, say this prayer."
1850 A.D.—"That prayer is superstition, drink this potion."
1940 A.D.—"That potion is snake oil, swallow this pill."
1985 A.D.—"That pill is ineffective, take this antibiotic."
2000 A.D.—"That antibiotic is artificial. Here, eat this root."

Anonymous

2

Hippocrates of Cos: The Most Famous Physician

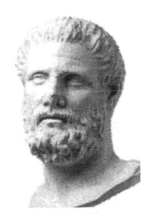

Hippocrates

Ancient Greek mythology told of Asklepios the great healer. The God Apollo and a mortal named Coronis had a son named Asklepios. Coronis was unfaithful and Artemis, the sister of Apollo, killed Coronis with her bow and arrow. Just before Coronis died, Apollo rescued his unborn son by cutting him from the womb of Coronis. Asklepios there received his name meaning "to cut open." The Centaur named Cherion raised him. Asklepios had a daughter named Panacea (universal cure), a daughter named Hygeia (health and beauty), and two sons who were battle surgeons. Asklepios became a great healer. He was so good that Hades, the god of the underworld, complained that not enough people were dying so he demanded that Zeus kill Asklepios. With his mighty thunderbolt Zeus did as his brother Hades requested. However, the Fates returned Asklepios to Mount Olympus and Asklepios became deified as the god of healing.

On the Island of Cos off the southwest coast of Turkey, a sect called Asklepiads worshiped Asklepios and practiced mystical religious-based teachings in temples devoted to him. The snake was felt to be sacred and the priests interpreted the dreams of the patients. Unlike the priests, the lay healers outside the temples used observation of results in their practice and had strong family traditions. In 460 B.C., Hippocrates was born into such an Asklepiad family. Hippocrates disassociated medicine from religious mysticism. He crystallized the existing knowledge into a systemic science. He was also the first to make physicians realize their high moral obligations to their patients.

Hippocratic physicians believed that nature needs to maintain equilibrium and if anything is out of balance disease results. They thought there were four fluids, or humors, that were the cause of certain emotions and behaviors: blood, yellow bile, black bile, and phlegm. Blood imparted energy, while yellow bile was choleric and made one quick to anger. Black bile was melancholic and introverted, and phlegm meant the brain was quiet and relaxed. Balance was health and an imbalance was the cause of disease. Because they kept accurate records of observations, this allowed them to make predictions or give a prognosis to the patient, and their reputation grew and grew.

Ptolemy I collected the entire medical works of the Hippocratic physicians under one title the *Corpus Hippocraticum*. In 1525, Pope Clement the VII compiled the first complete printed edition, which contained 70 different texts and was made up of writings before and after the death of Hippocrates. This work details the use of observation and record keeping, as well as the removal from medicine the notion of the supernatural. Also included is the famous Hippocratic Oath, which was the first ethical code of conduct for physicians. By swearing the Oath, the physician promised to hold his teacher as important as his parents, to teach his sons the art, and to keep his patients from harm. He swears that he will give no deadly drug, perform no abortion, and that he will not cut for stone. He also swears to visit the patient for their benefit only and to not have sex with the patient. Finally, he vows to keep matters confidential and act in a moral way. Some form of this oath is still taken by a great majority of doctors graduating from medical school today. Hippocrates remains the most famous and well-known physician even now some 2,500 years after his death.

"Life is short, the Art is long, opportunity is fleeting, experience is delusive, and judgment is difficult."

Hippocrates of Cos

3

Mythology and Medicine: The Symbol of Medicine

The symbol of Asklepios was his staff. The staff was a single knotty rod with a single serpent entwined about it, often with a Hippocratic saying.

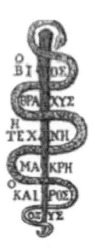

The origin of the staff is probably related to a practice of the Jews in the desert who would occasionally accidentally step on the parasite named *Drancunulus Medinensis,* a one and a half foot long worm. They removed the worm through the wound in the foot by wrapping it around a stick. Also the shedding of the skin by the snake symbolized the process of renewal and regeneration.

The caduceus, which is often thought to be the symbol of medicine, is two serpents entwined on a staff with wings at its top.

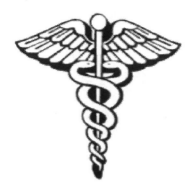

The caduceus is really the symbol of Hermes (Roman name— Mercury). Hermes was the winged foot messenger of the Gods and the symbol of commerce. A Swiss printer of medical books, Johan Froben, always used the caduceus on his frontispiece and so it became associated with medical books. The United States Military Corps mistakenly adopted the caduceus as its symbol in 1902 at the insistence of a single officer. Currently 70% of medical companies use the caduceus and 40% of medical professionals do as well.

The symbol of medicine is the staff of Asclepius *not* the caduceus.

"Good surgical judgment comes from bad experiences. Wisdom then comes from the experience of bad surgical judgment."

Anonymous

4

Mythology and Medicine: Achilles and Medusa

The Heel of Achilles

The Achilles tendon is the tendinous extension of the two calf muscles in the lower leg: the gastrocnemius and the soleus. The tendon passes posterior to the ankle. It is the thickest and strongest tendon in the body. It is about six inches long, and is inserted into the middle part of the posterior surface of the heel bone, the calcaneus.

The term *Achilles heel* is a deadly weakness, either literal or figurative that in spite of overall strength can potentially lead to downfall. The mythological term suggests a specific physical vulnerability, while today the term is used as a metaphor for attributes that can lead to failure. For example, "His pride was his Achilles heel."

Achilles was a Greek hero who was the central figure in Homer's *Iliad*. His mother Thetis wanted to make her baby son immortal and invulnerable so she held him by the heel and dipped him into the river Styx. The river Styx surrounded Hades and was the boundary between Earth and the Underworld (Hell). The Trojan named Paris killed Achilles. Paris shot an arrow that struck Achilles in the heel, his only vulnerable spot, and the great warrior Achilles died as a result of the injury.

The Head of Medusa

Medusa was a beautiful maiden who was the only mortal of the three sisters known as the Gorgons. One story has it that she lived far in the North and wanted to see the sun. She asked the goddess Athena for permission to visit the South and see the sun, but Athena refused. Medusa became angry and told Athena the reason she had refused her was that Athena was jealous of her beauty. Athena became incensed and punished Medusa by turning her hair into snakes and made her so ugly that anyone who looked upon her turned into stone.

Patients with cirrhosis of the liver can have increased resistance to blood flow through the portal vein, which increases the portal venous pressure. Portal hypertension then causes the portal venous blood to be shunted away from the liver into the systemic veins of the abdominal wall. These veins become engorged with blood, dilated, and appear as large varicosities around the umbilicus. They resemble the snakes on the head of Medusa. *Caput* is the Latin word meaning head. So the presence of dilated veins around the umbilicus is indicative of portal hypertension and is called the caput Medusa, or the head of Medusa.

"Abdominal Surgery—It is safer to look and see than to wait and see."

Sidney Cuthbert Wallace

5

The Barber Surgeon and the Barber Pole

In Medieval Europe surgery was not generally done by physicians, but by barbers. During the early Middle Ages, most healing arts (both medical and surgical), were practiced by members of the clergy. However, concern arose about the shedding of blood by these religious men and the Pope decreed that monks and priests should not and could not perform surgery. Therefore, the barbers who had experience with razors, in cutting the monks' hair, were chosen to perform the operations. The academic and social status of these barber-surgeons was much lower than that of physicians. Medicine was considered a profession practiced by doctors trained at a university. Surgery was a trade, sometimes carried out by the uneducated lower class.

Around the 13th century, guilds of barber-surgeons began appearing in Europe. In London, separate trade guilds for barbers and surgeons began as early as 1308, the two largest being the Company of Barbers (later known as the Barber-Surgeons' Company), and the much smaller but better educated Fellowship of Surgeons.

At the end of the fifteenth century, the two guilds had begun to work together on the licensing of surgeons, and in 1540 an act of Parliament combined the two guilds into one. They made certain laws, one of which prohibited surgeons from practicing as barbers and barbers from practicing surgery, with the one exception of the pulling of teeth. This association endured for two hundred years. It was ended in the 18th-century by surgeons across northern Europe who began to disassociate from their hair-cutting colleagues.

In 1745, London surgeons formed their own Company of Surgeons, which would evolve into the Royal College of Surgeons of England. As an interesting and lasting vestige of their history, today throughout the United Kingdom, surgeons are referred to as "Mister" and physicians are called "Doctor."

The red and white barber pole was associated with bloodletting and represented blood soaked bandages wrapped around a pole. The original poles had washbasins at the top and bottom: the leeches were placed in the upper basin and the bottom basin received the blood. The actual pole was the staff that the patient held onto during the bloodletting procedure. The United Barber Surgeons Company in England required a blue and white pole to be used by the barbers, and surgeons were required to use a red and white pole. Some would say the red of the barber pole represents arterial blood, the blue represents venous blood, and the white depicts the bandage.

"The fact that you do not know what to do does not mean that you have to do something."

Anonymous

6

The Patron Saints of Surgery

A patron saint is a saint who intercedes for the needs of their special charges. Many people know that the patron saint of travelers is Saint Christopher. Everyone knows the patron saint of lovers is Saint Valentine. The patron saint of Ireland is Saint Patrick and the patron saint of children visits every December 25th as Saint Nicholas. But who is the patron saint of surgeons?

Twin brothers Cosmos and Damian were the youngest of five brothers and were born in present day Turkey in the 3rd century A.D. They practiced the art of healing in Agea and then Syria. They accepted no payment for their services and because of this were called the *unmercenary* and attracted many to the Christian faith. They were arrested under the persecution of Christians by Diocletian and ordered to recant their faith. When they refused, they were crucified, shot with arrows, and beheaded. They were canonized for their miraculous cures—the most famous being transplantation of the leg of an Ethiopian onto a Christian Roman deacon with a malignant growth. They were the patron saints of the Medici family in Florence. Their feast day is September 26 and their major shrine is the Basilica of Saints Cosmos and Damian in Bari, Italy. So the patron saints of surgeons are Cosmos and Damian.

"To eliminate that which is superfluous, restore that which has been dislocated, separate that which has been united, join that which has been divided and repair the defects of nature."

Ambrose Paré

7

A Brief History of Cesarean Section

C esarean section is mentioned in the works of almost all
ancient cultures and folklore. As mentioned earlier, the
Greek god Apollo removed his son Asclepius from his mother's
abdomen. The Roman book of Laws named *Lex Caesarea* required
that the child be cut from the womb of a mother who died in
childbirth. Religious edicts of the time required that the mother
not be buried pregnant. The mother and the baby were buried
in separate graves. This practice then became a way to save the
baby. This measure of last resort was for the baby and not done to
save the mother's life. The ability to save both the mother and the
child would not become a routine possibility until the middle of
the nineteenth century. The notion that the name *Cearean section*
refers to the manner of birth of the Roman emperor Julius Caesar
is false. Cesarean sections were performed in Roman times to
save the baby but there are no writings that document a mother
surviving such a delivery. Caesar's mother was alive to serve him
as an advisor when he was emperor.

The first written record of a mother and baby surviving a
Cesarean section was from Switzerland in 1500 when Jacob Nufer,
a pig gelder, performed the operation on his wife. Mrs. Nufer would
go on to give birth normally to five children, including twins. The
child delivered by Cesarean section lived to the ripe old age of 77.
However, some seriously doubt the accuracy of this story.

The first successful Cesarean section in the United States of
America occurred in Mason County, Virginia in 1794. Dr. Jesse

Bennett performed the procedure on his wife Elizabeth. After the development of anesthesia, antisepsis, and asepsis, obstetricians began to improve the techniques employed in cesarean section.

In 1882, Max Saumlnger of Leipzig published his report on uterine sutures. This paper had a major impact on the surgical technique of cesarean section. Saumlnger's paper was based largely on the experience of U.S. surgeons who had used internal sutures. He recommended the new silver wire sutures developed by J. Marion Sims. The use of a transverse incision to minimize bleeding was also an advance that improved the outcomes of Cesarean section.

The rate of cesarean section in developed countries recommended by the World Health Organization is between 10% and 15% of all births.

In Italy, the incidence of Cesarean sections is particularly high and averages about 45%.

In the United States, the Cesarean rate has doubled since 1996, reaching a level of 31.8% in 2007. China has the highest rates of cesarean sections in the world at almost 50% in 2008.

The high rate of c-sections can be attributed to several reasons, such as medical malpractice concerns, the controversy surrounding the safety of vaginal birth after c-section, mothers' wises, remuneration, convenience of both the obstetrician and the patient, and concern over body image.

However, two things cannot be denied: the operation has saved countless lives of both mother and baby, and the name is from a book of Roman law named after Caesar and, unlike Shakespeare's character Macduff, not because Julius Caesar was born by being "from his mother's womb untimely ripped."

"Let the sun never set or rise on a small bowel obstruction."
Georg Friedrich Louis Stromeyer

8

Andreas Vesalius:
Human Anatomy Redefined

If Hippocrates is the most famous physician, then Claudius Galen would be the second most influential physician in history. Galen was born in 129 A.D. and became the surgeon to the Roman Emperor Marcus Aurelius. Galen was proliferative in his writings and teachings, argumentative, and arrogant, as he proclaimed himself to be infallible. His voluminous writings were collected and published in 1525. He only dissected animals; therefore, his teachings included many mistakes in human anatomy. But because of his status and writings, whatever Galen said was taken as the ultimate truth for fifteen centuries! It took the most famous anatomy book in history to correct Galen and redefine the discipline of human anatomy.

Andreas Vesalius was born on Christmas Eve in Brussels in 1514. He studied at the University of Paris and there he was taught Galenic anatomy. He later became a Professor of Anatomy at Padua, Italy. He dissected human cadavers and had the courage to correct Galen's inaccurate anatomical descriptions.

In 1543, he wrote his famous text entitled *De Humani Coporis Fabrica.* There were seven volumes on the structure of the human body. Not only was the anatomy accurate, but Vesalius was also the first to actually describe how to properly dissect the human body. This text is regarded as a masterpiece in medicine, but it is also a masterpiece of art. The numerous anatomical illustrations are anatomically perfect and in classic Italian renaissance style. Stephan Von Kalkar, a student of the Titian school, was the artist.

After the publication of his book, Vesalius was invited to be the personal physician to the Emperor Charles V. In 1564, he went on a pilgrimage to the Holy Land. On his return trip, he was shipwrecked on a Greek island and died at the age of fifty.

"The doctor is nature's assistant."

Claudius Galen

9

William Harvey:
The Circulation of Blood Described

Just as Vesalius corrected Galenic anatomy, Harvey corrected Galen's theory of the circulation of the blood. Galen recognized the difference between venous or dark blood and arterial or light blood. He believed in a unidirectional system of circulation. Galen proclaimed that venous blood was produced by the liver and then consumed by all organs of the body and similarly arterial blood was made in the heart and consumed by all organs.

Harvey's little book entitled De *Motu Cordis* (usually referred to as *"On the Motion of the Heart and Blood"*) corrected Galen and proved the systemic circulation of the blood.

William Harvey was born in Folkstone, England in 1578. After graduating from college in Cambridge, he went on to study medicine at the University of Padua in Italy. He returned to Cambridge and received an M.D. degree from there as well. In 1609, he accepted a position as physician in charge at Saint Bartholomew's Hospital in London where he stayed for the rest of his life.

In 1628 he published his famous 72 page book, *Exercitatio Anatomica de Motu Cordis et Sanguinis in Animalibus*, commonly referred to as "de Motu Cordis."

Galen believed that the liver was the origin of venous blood. Harvey estimated how much blood is expelled with each beat of the heart and the number of times the heart beats in half an hour. All of these estimates were kept low to increase acceptance. He estimated that the capacity of the heart was 1.5 ounces (43 ml), and that the heart delivers 1/8 of that amount blood with each beat. Harvey estimated that about $\frac{1}{6}$ ounces (4.7 ml) of blood went through the heart every time it beat and that since the heart beats about a 1000 times every half hour, it would have to pump 10 pounds 6 ounces of blood in half an hour. Therefore, the liver would have to make more than 500 pounds of blood in a day. Clearly Galen was wrong. Harvey then proved a single circuit of blood flow by animal experiments that included tying off the arteries and seeing the heart enlarge, then tying off the veins and watching the heart empty.

Harvey went on to become the physician to King James I and then King Charles I. He retired at age 68 and died twelve years later at the age of 80 from what was probably a cerebral hemorrhage.

"All we know is still infinitely less than all that remains unknown."

William Harvey

10

A History of General Anesthesia

E arly anesthetics were called soporifics. A soporific dulls the senses or produces sleep. Narcotics were also used to help relieve pain. The ancient Romans used opium and a variety of plants that contained potent alkaloids such as jimson weed, marijuana, and belladonna. Other early techniques used included alcohol, acupuncture, ice, and hypnosis. Ancient Incas produced a local anesthetic effect by chewing cocoa leaves and spitting into the wound.

By the middle of the nineteenth century, the two agents most often used were alcohol and opiates. Both had serious side effects and neither had the desired outcome of completely alleviating pain.

A Swiss physician named Paracelus used a flammable chemical liquid called "sweet vitriol" on chickens. He reported that when the chickens breathed the gas they not only fell asleep, but they also felt no pain. In 1730, a German chemist named Frobenius gave the liquid the name we know it by today—ether. The word *ether* is taken from the Greek meaning pure air.

In 1772, Joseph Priestly discovered the gas nitrous oxide and described how to produce it. A few years later, in Bristol, England, a chemist named Humphrey Davy discovered that inhaling nitrous oxide made him laugh and so he called it "laughing gas." By the early 19th century, laughing gas parties were commonplace. In December of 1844, a Hartford, Connecticut dentist named Horace Wells went to a public demonstration of nitrous oxide and when he witnessed a participant injure his knee and feel no pain,

Wells thought of the potential anesthetic use of the gas. Then he persuaded a colleague to pull one of his teeth while he was breathing nitrous oxide and he too, experienced no pain. Wells traveled to Boston to describe his discovery to a former student of his, William T.G. Morton. Morton convinced the famous Massachusetts General Hospital surgeon John Collins Warren to try surgery with the use of inhalational nitrous oxide as an anesthetic. In January of 1845, Wells administered nitrous oxide for Warren as he operated on a schoolboy in front of a Harvard medical school class. The boy cried out in pain, Warren called nitrous oxide a "humbug" and Wells was disgraced.

Then Charles Jackson, a dentist and former classmate of Morton, suggested that sulfuric ether be used instead of nitrous oxide. On October 16, 1846, in a surgical amphitheater now called the "Ether Dome," at the Massachusetts General Hospital in Boston, John Collins Warren removed a tumor from the jaw of Edward Abbott and the patient had no pain or memory of the operation. Warren declared, "Gentleman, this is no humbug," and the modern era of surgery had begun.

Wells, Jackson, and Morton each claimed to be the inventor of general anesthesia. Wells, disgraced by his failure, went on to give up dentistry and became a travelling salesman. He soon became addicted to chloroform. He then went on to alcohol and in New York City while intoxicated by both, threw sulfuric ether on two prostitutes. He was arrested and jailed. While in jail he committed suicide.

Morton read an article in the *Atlantic Journal* that supported Jackson as the inventor of anesthesia. He became so upset that he had a stroke and died. Jackson, after visiting Morton's gravesite where he read the headstone that proclaimed Morton to be the inventor of anesthesia, went insane and had to be institutionalized for the remaining seven years of his life.

"It takes five years to learn when to operate and twenty more to learn when not to."

Anonymous

11

The First Use of Ether for Surgical Anesthesia

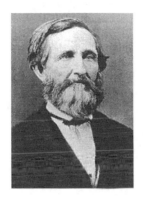

Crawford Williamson Long

(Public Domain Copyright Expired)

C rawford Williamson Long was born on November 1, 1815, in Danielsville, Georgia. He was the son of a wealthy merchant and cousin of the infamous John Henry "Doc" Holliday. At the young age of fourteen he entered the University of Georgia in Athens, Georgia. There his roommate was Alexander Stephens, the future vice president of the Confederacy during the Civil War. After graduating in 1835, he started his medical education at Transylvania College in Lexington, Kentucky, but left after one year, transferring to the University of Pennsylvania in Philadelphia. It was there he obtained his medical degree in 1839. In 1841, after a hospital internship in New York City, Long returned to Jefferson, Georgia to begin his practice of medicine and surgery.

During his medical school years, Long had seen laughing gas parties and "ether frolics," and noticed that those who would inhale laughing gas or sulfuric ether felt no pain until the effects of the gases were gone. He performed his first surgical procedure using sulfuric ether on March 30, 1842, when he excised a tumor from the neck of a young man. Long continued to use sulfuric ether as an anesthetic but did not publish his efforts. Long read about William Morton who used sulfuric ether as an anesthetic, which prompted him to publish his use of it in the *Southern Medical and Surgical Journal* in 1849. Although he used ether several years ahead of the others in Boston, Long would not get full credit for this major advance in surgery until after his death.

In 1851, Long and his wife Caroline moved to Athens, Georgia where he joined his brother Robert in practice. During the Civil War he remained in Athens and treated both Union and Confederate soldiers. He died in Athens, Georgia on June 16, 1878.

Although William Morton is well known for his role in the discovery of anesthesia on October 16, 1846 in Boston, Massachusetts, Crawford W. Long was the first to have used ether-based anesthesia. Long is now recognized by medical societies worldwide and has been remembered in many ways including monuments, statues, and a U.S. postage stamp. Doctors' Day is celebrated every March 30th, which is the day that Long first used ether anesthesia. In 1931, the Davis-Fischer Sanatorium on Linden Avenue in Atlanta, Georgia was renamed Crawford W. Long Memorial Hospital in honor of Dr. Long. In February of 2009, the now 500—bed teaching hospital was renamed Emory University Hospital Midtown, but the original name is maintained on its exterior monuments. A statue of Dr. Crawford Long stands in the United States Capitol as one of the two monuments to representing the state of Georgia.

"There are two groups of surgeons, those who see what they believe, and those who believe what they see."

Owen H. Wangensteen, MD

12

Wash Your Hands

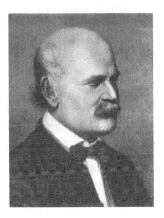

Ignaz Phillip Semmelweis
(Copper plate engraving by Jenő Doby Public Domain, Copyright expired)

C hildbed fever, or puerperal fever is a bacterial infection
seen in women following childbirth or miscarriage, and
was common in the early nineteenth century. The mortality rate
for these women was as high as 35% in some institutions. One
young doctor came to find a way to save the women, but in so
doing lost his career and his life.

The son of a Hungarian grocer, Ignaz Phillip Semmelweis
(1818-1865) began his study of law in 1837. He then switched
his career to the study of medicine, entering the University
of Vienna, and graduating in 1844. He decided to practice

obstetrics and gained a position as house surgeon at the Vienna General Hospital. One of Semmelweis's colleagues and good friend at the hospital was dissecting a cadaver while teaching medical students and was cut with the knife. He developed an overwhelming infection and died. Semmelweis realized that his friend's autopsy findings were the same as the women who had died from puerperal fever. He thought that some cadaverous material must be responsible for the infection. This would explain why the women who delivered in the midwives' clinic had such a lower rate of childbed fever than those women delivered in the medical students' clinic. The medical students and physicians would come directly from the autopsy room to the delivery room, thereby passing on the contamination and causing the deaths of the women. The midwives were not allowed in the autopsy room. He realized that the contaminated hands of the physicians were causing the problem. The answer had to be to clean the hands of the doctors before they administered to the patients. He instituted a strict policy of hand washing followed by cleaning the hands with a chlorinated lime solution. The results of the hand washing policy were immediate and dramatic. The mortality rate was cut by 90%!

However, the doctors didn't like the chlorinated lime solution as it irritated the hands; they felt there was no known reason as to why it should be effective, and so they resisted. Semmelweis became irritated and publically denounced their "ignorance". Soon Semmelweis' superiors had had enough of the controversy and his demeanor, and his contract was not renewed. He then took a position in a Budapest hospital, and once again the mortality rate from childbed fever was drastically reduced. He published his results but when his writings were met with apathy and disbelief, he became increasingly irritable and depressed, and turned to alcohol and prostitutes. His concerned family had him placed in a mental hospital. He became so distraught he was placed in a straitjacket and housed in a ward for violent patients. He tried to escape and was beaten by the guards, suffering many cuts and bruises. He developed multiple wound infections and died just two weeks after being placed in the asylum. He was forty-seven years old. His theories died with him, but he would much later get the credit he deserved as a savior of pregnant women.

"The dextrous hand must not be allowed to reach before imperfect judgment."

Sir Zachary Cope

13

The Birth of the Germ Theory and Bacteriology

L ouis Pasteur (December 27, 1822-September 28, 1895) was a French chemist and microbiologist born in Dole, France. He is probably best known for his discovery of a method of preventing milk and wine from spoilage and souring. That process today is called pasteurization. He also invented the first vaccine for rabies. His work formed the basis for the germ theory of disease. He and Robert Koch are generally considered to be the fathers of microbiology.

Prior to Pasteur it was generally believed that certain organisms such as maggots could spontaneously arise from dead flesh or fleas could arise from dust in the air. Pasteur demonstrated that fermentation is caused by the growth of microorganisms, and that the growth of those microorganisms is not due to spontaneous generation, as was previously believed, but rather is the result of the production of new living organisms from other living organisms. Living things come from other living things by reproduction. The Latin phrase *omne vivum ex vivo* (all life is from life) summarizes the germ theory and rejects spontaneous generation. Pasteur invented a process of heating milk and other liquids to kill the bacteria and molds already present in them.

This discovery led Pasteur to the theory that ever-present microorganisms could infect humans and cause disease. This theory led Joseph Lister to develop his antiseptic methods in surgery.

"Where observation is concerned, chance favors only the prepared mind."

Louis Pasteur

14

The Discovery of Antisepsis

Joseph Lister (1827-1895) was an English surgeon who discovered the antiseptic method. This giant step in the fight against postoperative infection set the stage for the beginning of modern surgery.

Joseph Lister was born in Upton, Essex, England, on April 5, 1827. Lister wanted to become a surgeon at a young age. He attended the University College in London, England, to study medicine. After graduating in 1852, he began a surgical career in Edinburgh, Scotland. When he was 26 years old he became a member of the Royal College of Surgeons. In 1854, he became the assistant to James Syme at the University of Scotland in Edinburgh. In 1860, he became professor of surgery at the Royal Infirmary in Glasgow, Scotland, and it was here that he became aware of Pasteur's work that led him to his work in reducing postoperative infections.

Although anesthesia had been introduced in the 1840's, the number of elective operations done did not increase because of the very high mortality rate associated with postoperative infections.

Lister's research was mainly concerned with the microscopic changes in tissue that result in inflammation. Lister proposed that heat, chemicals, or filtration were the ways to prevent the growth of bacteria that caused gangrene. When Lister became aware of Pasteur's work he concluded that inflammation was the result of germs entering and then developing in the wound.

Lister had read a report that in Carlisle, England the treatment of sewage with a chemical called carbolic acid had led to a reduction of diseases in both the people and among the cattle grazing on those sewage-treated fields. Lister sprayed carbolic acid onto surgical instruments, dressings, and even in the air of the operating room. He found that lint dressings soaked in carbolic acid greatly reduced the infection rate in open fractures. He required that surgeons wash their bloody coats and wash their hands with carbolic acid before and after the operation. Antisepsis became a basic principle of surgery. Amputations became less frequently required. Postoperative deaths from infections were greatly reduced.

In 1869 Lister returned to Edinburgh as the Syme professor of surgery. He later left Scotland and moved to London. He won worldwide acclaim, honors, and honorary doctorates, and he was made a baron in 1897. In 1879, Listerine mouthwash was named in his honor for his work in antisepsis.

He died at Walmer Hospital in Kent, England, on February 10, 1912.

"It has been said that there are only two periods in the history of surgery—before Lister and after Lister."

Harvey Graham

15

A Brief History Blood Transfusion

Early attempts at transfusing blood from one person into another were usually met with very poor results. Pope Innocent VIII (1432-1492) sank into a coma as physicians poured the blood from three young Italian boys into his mouth (the circulation of blood had not yet been discovered). The boys were paid a single ducat each. Pope Innocent VIII as well as the three boys died as a result of the attempt.

William Harvey described the circulatory system in 1628. In 1665, Richard Lower successfully transfused blood from one dog into another. The first successful animal to human transfusion occurred in 1667 when Jean-Baptiste Denis of France's Academie des sciences transfused lamb's blood into a human. Although this practice was sometimes successful, because of frequent human deaths after these transfusions, the Catholic Church issued general prohibitions against transfusion and it fell from orthodox medical practice for 150 years.

Dr. James Blundell did the first successful human-to-human blood transfusion at Guy's Hospital in London, England in 1818. Four ounces of blood was transfused from a man into his wife, who suffered from severe post-partum hemorrhage. The patient died but Blundell later transfused 10 additional patients, about half of whom survived. Early transfusions were risky and many resulted in the death of the patient.

Then in 1901, Karl Landsteiner discovered human blood groups, and this allowed for much safer blood transfusions. When blood is mixed from two incompatible individuals, an immune response occurs that results in the destruction or lysis of red blood cells. This breakdown of the red cell releases free hemoglobin into the bloodstream with potential fatal consequences. Landsteiner discovered that the clumping seen during mixture of incompatible blood types resulted from an immunological reaction due to the recipient's blood containing antibodies to the donor's blood. His work made it possible to determine the A, B, and O blood types and allowed a way for blood transfusions to be carried out much more safely. He was awarded the Nobel Prize in Physiology and Medicine in 1930. Blood transfusion during an operation was first accomplished at the Cleveland Clinic in Ohio in 1905. The surgeon was George Crile.

The transfusions described above were direct transfusions from donor to recipient. Attempts to store blood resulted in coagulation of the blood, rendering it useless. In 1914, it was found that the addition of anticoagulants to the blood allowed storage of the blood for later use. Then in the 1940's, the Rhesus blood group system (Rh+ and Rh-) was discovered. Shortly thereafter, the introduction of the acid-citrate-dextrose (ACD) solution reduced the volume of anticoagulant needed and allowed greater volumes of blood to be transfused. Longer-term storage was also made possible by ACD anticoagulation. Storage in plastic bags replaced the glass bottles in the 1950's.

In 1937, Bernard Fantus originated the term *blood bank* when he established the first hospital blood bank in the United States at the Cook County Hospital in Chicago, Illinois. The transfusion of blood and blood components ranks with anesthesia, antibiotics, parenteral nutrition, and X-rays as being among the greatest advances in the history of surgery.

"I firmly believe that the best possible operation is not the same thing as the best operation possible"

RodneySmith

16

The First Laparotomy

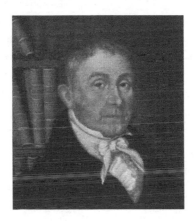

Ephraim McDowell
(Public Domain National Library of Medicine)

E phraim McDowell (1771-1830) was an American physician who was the first to successfully remove an ovarian tumor. McDowell was born in Rockbridge County, Virginia and moved to Danville, Kentucky. Although he spent three years as a medical student in Virginia, attended lectures in medicine at the University of Edinburgh, Scotland and studied privately with Dr. John Bell, he never got a medical degree. In 1795, he returned to Danville, Kentucky and began his practice as a surgeon. On December 13, 1809, Dr. McDowell travelled to Green County, Kentucky, sixty miles away, to see Jane Todd Crawford. McDowell diagnosed her as having an ovarian tumor and assured her that he would operate and make an effort to remove the tumor if only she would come to his home in Danville. She rode the sixty miles on horseback while balancing the tumor on the saddle horn.

It was on Christmas morning in 1809 when Dr. McDowell began the historic procedure. There was no anesthesia and no antisepsis, only the prayers of the family gathered outside and the sounds of the hymns Jane Crawford sang during her twenty five minute operation. The ovarian tumor weighed 22.5 pounds. Mrs. Crawford made a completely uncomplicated recovery and went back home to Green County three weeks after the operation. She lived another 32 years. This was the first successful removal of an ovarian tumor in the world. This historic operation was accomplished not by a Harvard professor or English lord, but by a surgeon in rural western Kentucky with no anesthesia, no sterile technique, no antibiotics, and no MD degree.

All attempts at any operation inside the abdominal cavity before McDowell's laparotomy had been met with death. McDowell did not publish an account of this historic operation until 1817, and by then he had performed two more similar procedures.

In June 1830 Dr. McDowell experienced an acute attack of severe abdominal pain, nausea, and fever. He died on June 25, most likely as a result of perforated appendicitis.

"Primum non nocere—first of all, do no harm."

Hippocrates

17

The First Gastrectomy

C hristian Albert Theodor Billroth (1829-1894) was an
Austrian surgeon who is best known for performing the
first gastrectomy. Billroth attended the University of Greisswald
to study medicine and then received his medical degree at the
University of Berlin. Billroth practiced in Berlin at the Charité
Medical University from 1853-1860. While in Berlin he was
an apprentice to Bernhard Von Langenbeck, who was known
as the father of European surgical residency training. Billroth
then moved on to become the director of the surgical clinic and
professor of surgery at the University of Zurich from 1860-1867.
In 1867, he became professor of surgery at the University
of Vienna, and the chief of the Second Surgical Clinic at the
Allgemeine Krankenhaus.

Billroth was responsible for many firsts in surgery. He
performed the first esophagectomy (1871), the first laryngectomy
(1873), and as stated above, the first successful gastrectomy
(1881) for gastric cancer. The patient was Ms. Therese Heller
who was 43 years old, bedridden, weak and emaciated. She
developed continual vomiting and had a palpable epigastric
mass. Billroth removed an obstructing prepyloric gastric cancer.
The reconstruction would be become known as a Billroth I
(gastroduodenostomy). Ms. Heller was able to take nourishment
on the first day following the surgery. She died 4 months later
and at autopsy was found to have widespread metastatic disease.

While in Zurich Billroth studied the viola and played in a string quartet. He met musician Johannes Brahms and they became close friends, corresponding with each other often. Brahms would often play his new compositions in Billroth's home before his public performances. Brahms even dedicated his first two string quartets to Billroth.

Billroth saw the art in the science of surgery as well as music. He wrote, "It is one of the superficialities of our time to see in science and in art two opposites. Imagination is the mother of both."

"The pleasure of a physician is little, the gratitude of patients is rare, and even rarer is material reward, but these things will never deter the student who feels the call within him."

Theodor Billroth

18

The History of Appendectomy

D r. Kurt Semm did the first laparoscopic appendectomy in 1981. Today, single incision laparoscopic surgery is being applied to appendectomy. There have been reports of appendectomy in humans by NOTES (Natural Orifice Transabdominal Endoscopic Surgery). In other words, the scope is passed through the stomach or vagina and the appendix is removed, and then the perforation of the stomach or vagina is closed leaving no visible skin incision. But how did we get here?

The ancient Greeks did not mention the appendix. Interestingly some have written that Hippocrates himself may have died of perforated appendicitis. Galen, the most famous Roman physician, who was the final word in medicine for 1,000 years, did not mention the appendix as he dissected only monkeys and did not dissect humans (or orangutans, chimpanzees, or wombats—the only species with an appendix). The appendix was first described in 1522 by Carpus of Padua, Italy. Vesalius then illustrated the appendix in 1543. Fallopius (of Fallopian tube fame) was the first to compare the appendix to a worm—*vermiform* appendix.

Abdominal pain above the umbilicus was termed iliac passion and was routinely treated with purgatives and bloodletting. Pain below the navel was termed colic passion and was treated with cathartics. Appendicitis led to perforation and death unless the abscess ruptured through the skin and caused an enterocutaneous fistula.

There was great debate over the cause of iliac passion in the right lower quadrant. It was called typhlitis (from the Greek *tuphlon* meaning caecum) or perithyplitis as it was felt to be inflammation of the caecum, which is the pouch like beginning of the large intestine. In 1886, Sir Reginald Fitz, a Harvard pathologist, showed that the symptoms of more than 200 hundred cases of typhlitis were identical to more than 200 cases of autopsy-proven perforated appendicitis. He was the first to use the term appendicitis and the first to state that the cause of the disease was the appendix and advocated its early removal. So, after Fitz, many doctors began to operate for appendicitis. In 1893, Dr. Charles McBurney described his muscle splitting incision still in use today for open procedures. One of the most famous cases of appendicitis and appendectomy was that of King Edward the VII, the first-born son of Queen Victoria. Two weeks before his scheduled coronation he developed appendicitis. When he wanted to refuse surgery so that he could go to his upcoming coronation, the famous surgeon Sir Fredrick Treves told him that without the surgery he would attend the coronation as a corpse. The future king relented and was operated on by Treves in a room at Buckingham Palace. He survived and went to his delayed coronation and ruled for 7 more years.

"The quality of the surgical care you receive is directly related to where you go to get it."

Alexander Paderewski

19

Advances in Appendectomy

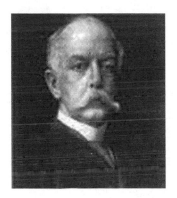

Charles McBurney
(Public Domain National Library of Medicine)

M cBurney's Point is a point 1/3 of the distance from
the right anterior superior iliac spine (ASIS) towards
the umbilicus. It is the point of maximal tenderness in acute
appendicitis. Every physician and medical student knows
McBurney's Point—but who was McBurney?

Charles McBurney was born in 1845. He graduated from
Harvard College in 1866, and received his degree as a doctor
of medicine from the College of Physicians and Surgeons of
Columbia University in New York. He interned at Bellevue
Hospital in New York and then went to Paris, Vienna, and London
for further training. In 1888, he was appointed surgeon-in-chief
of the Roosevelt Hospital in New York. It was at the Roosevelt

that he did his most famous work on appendicitis. He described McBurney's Point and also his muscle splitting incision that surgeons still utilize today. McBurney loved to hunt and fish. In 1913, while on a hunting trip, he suffered a heart attack and died at age 68.

"More is missed by not looking than by not knowing."
Anonymous

20

Pancreaticoduodenectomy

A llen Oldfather Whipple (1881-1963) was an American surgeon who is known for an operation that is performed to treat pancreatic cancer.

Whipple was born in Azerbaijan, Persia (modern day Iran). He attended Princeton University in 1904, and received his M.D. from the Columbia University College of Physicians and Surgeons in 1908. He completed two years of postgraduate work at Roosevelt Hospital in New York City. He became professor of surgery at Columbia University and operated there for twenty-five years. In 1931, the Valentine Mott chair of surgery was established for him. It was during his time at Columbia that he developed the procedure for resection of the pancreas (pancreaticoduodenectomy) now known as the "Whipple procedure." Since his original description, there have been significant modifications of his technique. Whipple performed 37 pancreaticoduodenectomies during his career. When it became known that some patients could be cured of their hypoglycemic symptoms by removing an insulinoma from the pancreas, Whipple developed a set of criteria for operating to look for pancreatic insulinoma:

1) symptoms known or likely to be caused by hypoglycemia,
2) a low plasma glucose measured at the time of the symptoms, and
3) relief of symptoms when the glucose is raised to normal. These criteria came to be known as Whipple's Triad.

He retired in 1946 as professor emeritus and consultant in surgery.

Whipple became president of the American College of Physicians and Surgeons. He was trustee of Princeton University and received the 1958 Woodrow Wilson Award. He spoke several languages and was an authority on ancient cultures and literature. He died at age 82 in Princeton, New Jersey.

"It is much more important to know what sort of a patient has a disease than what sort of a disease a patient has."

William Osler

21

The First Perineal Prostatectomy

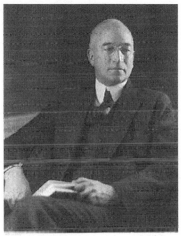

Hugh Hampton Young
(Public Domain US Copyright Expired)

H ugh Hampton Young, MD (1870-1945) was born in San
Antonio, Texas on September 18, 1870. He was the son
of Confederate Brigadier General William Hugh Young. When
he was 21 years old, Young graduated from the University of
Virginia in 1891 after acquiring a BA, MA, and MD degrees in just
four years. In 1895 he began teaching at Johns Hopkins Institute.
At the age of 27, he was the first head of the new department of
urology. He would remain at Johns Hopkins until 1940.

In 1903, having developed the operation of perineal prostatectomy for the relief of bladder-outlet obstruction, Young examined two patients in whom the size of prostatic cancer was small. He wrote that he thought that it would be possible to cure these patients if the entire prostate and its capsule could be removed. He made sketches of his plan for prostatectomy and showed them to his famous chief of surgery Dr. William S. Halsted. Halsted encouraged him to continue his work. In April of 1904, with the assistance of Halsted, he performed the first radical perineal prostatectomy for cancer of the prostate.

Among Young's contributions to medicine are several inventions and discoveries, primarily relating to surgery. Besides several surgical instruments, he and his associates also discovered the antiseptic merbromin, more popularly known as Mercurochrome.

He died in August of 1945 at the age of 74 and is buried in Baltimore, Maryland.

"Surgeons must be very careful
When they take the knife!
Underneath their fine incisions
Stirs the Culprit—Life!"

Emily Dickinson

22

The Use of Rubber Gloves in Surgery

William Stewart Halsted, the first Chairman of the Department of Surgery at Johns Hopkins Hospital in Baltimore, operated barehanded like every other surgeon in the world. Dr. Halsted followed the antiseptic principles of Lister and used carbolic acid and mercuric chloride to disinfect the hands of the operating personnel. Caroline Hampton, his operating room nurse, developed dermatitis from the chemicals. Halstead wrote, "As she was an unusually efficient woman, I gave the matter my consideration." In 1890, he asked the Goodyear Rubber Company to manufacture two pairs of thin rubber gloves with gauntlets that could withstand the carbolic acid. Within a few years, every member of the operating team at Johns Hopkins wore thin rubber gloves during operative procedures. However, widespread use of rubber gloves in the operating room did not uniformly occur until after World War I.

Caroline Hampton was the niece of the famous Confederate General Wade Hampton. He would later become the governor of South Carolina and then a United States senator. Dr. Halsted married Caroline Hampton in 1890. They had no children. The Halsteds vacationed for four months every year at their home in the mountains near Cashiers, North Carolina. They both died in 1922. The home and surrounding 2000 acres were sold and eventually became the High Hampton Inn and Country Club, which is still in operation today. Halsted's picture hangs, without fanfare, in the dining room.

"Never let the skin stand in the way of a diagnosis."

Anonymous

23

The White Coat

White coats have been seen as the distinguishing garment of doctors for more than a century. However, before the great advances of the late 19th century, the practice of medicine was not held in high regard by the public. A visit from the doctor was often a part of the dying process and was not a welcomed event. With the advances in science such as Lister's ideas of antisepsis and the discovery of anesthesia, there came a greater respect for those using science to heal. Surgeons now understood anatomy, could arrest blood loss, control pain, and operate with a much lower chance of infection. By the end of the 19th century the chance of dying after surgery had gone from over 40% to about 10%, depending on the operation. The "whiteness" or "pureness" of medicine was then displayed in the dress of physicians and nurses. The word *candor* means truth and openness and is derived from the Latin *candida*, which means "pure white."

Before the late 19th century, physicians, as well as the clergy, dressed in black. Black attire was, and is, considered formal and indicates the seriousness and solemnity of the wearer. Students who were examining cadavers would even wear black lab coats in an effort to indicate their respect for what was the person they were dissecting. With the advances in the science of medicine, physicians wanted to be seen more as scientists and began to wear the white laboratory coat of the scientist.

A recent study conducted in the United Kingdom found that the majority of patients prefer their doctors to wear white coats; however, most doctors prefer less formal clothing, such as scrubs. The physician in a white coat has become one of the lasting symbols of the medical profession. But the white coat has also become such an intimidating symbol that some pediatricians and psychiatrists generally choose not to wear it in order to reduce the anxiety level in their patients.

Most medical schools now observe the entrance of a new class with a white coat ceremony. The white coat ceremony originated in Columbia University's College of Physicians and Surgeons in 1993 and involves a ceremonial putting of the white coat on the student by the professor. Most medical students and residents in training are traditionally required by their institution to wear short white coats, and the long white coat is reserved for the attending physician who has completed training.

"Nothing ruins surgical research like good follow up."

B. Raman

24

The History of Surgical Attire

Until well into the 20th century, surgeons wore their street clothes into the operating room. They wore no mask or head cover and operated barehanded without gloves. The amount of dried blood on his coat was a source of pride that bespoke how busy the surgeon was.

But after Lister, surgeons hung up their operating coats and started wearing clean operating gowns and gauze masks during surgery. The mask was not to protect the patient but to protect the surgeon from contamination by the patient. As detailed in the previous chapter, rubber gloves came into the operating room at about the same time. Once again, these were worn to protect the hands from the carbolic acid and mercuric acid and not to protect the patient.

Medical science's understanding of the causes of wound infection brought about the use of antiseptic linen drapes and gowns in the operating room. By the 1940s, all of the instruments and supplies were routinely steam or gas sterilized.

Originally, operating room attire was white, but an all-white environment led to eyestrain for both the surgeon and staff. By the 1960s, most hospitals had adopted various shades of green or blue for operating room clothing and drapes, which provided a softer visual environment and reduced eye fatigue.

Most hospitals now use different colored scrub suits to differentiate between the different hospital departments, or different roles within the operating room suite. Non-clinical personnel and medical device sales representatives are often identified by a distinct color of scrub attire.

Also beginning in the 1940s it became standard for all operating room personnel to wear caps or bouffant hats to cover all hair and facial hair. Since the 1970s, standard surgical attire has included a short-sleeve V-neck pull on shirt and drawstring pants. The hair is covered by a paper or cloth tie-back or bouffant-style cap, a cloth or synthetic surgical gown, latex gloves and closed-toe shoes covered with paper shoe covers.

"A chance to cut is a chance to cure, but the surgeon's work may be far from complete."

Anonymous

25

The History of the "Scrub Tech"

During World War I and World War II, the military used medics to work under the direct supervision of the surgeon. Also, the navy used medical corpsmen aboard combat ships. At that time, in the United States military, female nurses were prohibited from being on the battlefield or aboard combat ships. These medics and corpsmen led to a specialty within the military medical services called Operating Room Technicians (ORTs).

When there were shortages of operating room nurses in the civilian sector, hospitals began to recruit ex-medics and ex-corpsmen. At first these ex-military men functioned as the circulating nurse role in the operating room while the scrub, or instrument nurse, role continued to be performed by the registered nurse. In the mid-1960s the roles were reversed, and the ex-medic became the instrument nurse or Operating Room Technician.

In 1968, the American Association of Operating Room Nurses (AORN) developed the Association of Operation Room Technicians (AORT). Those candidates who passed the certification examination were given a new title: certified operating room technician (CORT). In 1973 AORT became independent of AORN and changed their name to the Association of Surgical Technologists (AST). Today, surgical technologists passing the national certification examination are given the title of certified surgical atechnologist (CST).

About 75% of the jobs for surgical technologists are in hospitals and ambulatory surgery centers and are mainly in operating and delivery rooms. Some technologists, known as private scrub techs, are hired and work directly for the surgeon.

"Life is short, art long, opportunity fleeting, experience misleading, and judgment difficult."

Hippocrates of Cos

26

The History of Surgery on the Mayo Stand

M ost of the instruments used in the operating room today carry the names of the famous surgeons that helped to develop them. Most of those names of these eponymous tools that are spoken in every operating room every day have been uttered by generations of operating room nurses and surgeons for over a hundred years. They are indeed the tools of the surgeon's trade. If you are a surgeon who calls out for them every day, their history should be of interest.

The Bard-Parker Scalpel: Early scalpels were made of a variety of substances including everything from wood and ivory to intricately carved tortoise shell handles. After Lister and the application of antiseptic techniques, these gave way to a single piece metal handle and blade. These required constant sharpening. In 1904, Mr. King Gillette patented the single and double-edged razor blade. These blades were placed in specialized holders or used by gripping them with surgical clamps. Morgan Parker invented and patented a two-piece scalpel with the blade and handle held together by metal parts. His design allowed for exchanging the old blade for a new one. He got together with Charles Russell Bard of the Bard Company and formed The Bard-Parker Company. The now ubiquitous Bard-Parker scalpel was born. Parker bought out Bard in 1923.

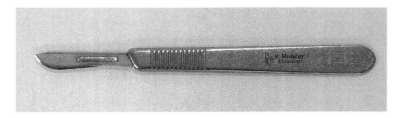

Bard-Parker Scalpel
(original photograph K. Roeder)

Kelly Clamp: Howard Atwood Kelly (1858-1943) was the first Chairman of Gynecology at Johns Hopkins Hospital and was a contemporary of Halstead and Osler. He established gynecology as a specialty.

He died at age 84 in Baltimore, Maryland, and his wife of 53 years died six hours later in the room next to his.

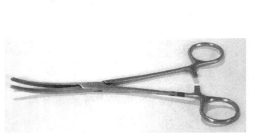

The Kelly Clamp
(original photograph K. Roeder)

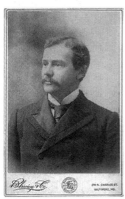

Howard Atwood Kelly
(Public Domain Copyright Expired)

Allis Forceps: Oscar Huntington Allis (1826-1921) was an orthopedic surgeon who graduated from Jefferson Medical College in Philadelphia. He is known for the Allis Sign which is a clinical sign associated with fracture of the hip, but most recognize his name by the toothed forceps he developed that are in every general surgery instrument set.

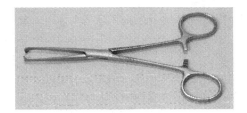

Allis Forceps
(original photograph K. Roeder)

Metzenbaum Scissors: Myron Firth Metzenbaum (1876-1944) practiced otolaryngology in Cleveland. He used the dissecting scissors he invented to remove inflamed tonsils. He was a student of the famous George Crile. He did not get a patent on his scissors and they are called "Mao Tse Tung Scissors" in China and "Mahatma Gandhi Scissors" in India.

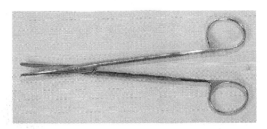

(original photograph K. Roeder)

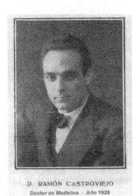

D. RAMÓN CASTROVIEJO
Doctor en Medicina - Año 1928

Ramon Castroviejo
(Public Domain Copyright expired)

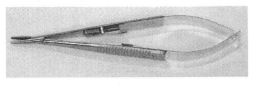

Castroviejo Needle Holder
(original photograph K. Roeder)

Castroviejo Needle Holder

Ramon Castroviejo (1904-1987) grew up in Spain but came to the United States to the Mayo Clinic. He eventually spent most of his professional years in New York. He was Chief of Ophthalmology at St. Vincent's Hospital there. He perfected the technique of corneal transplant. He developed roughly sixty instruments in his career, including the needle holder that bears his name.

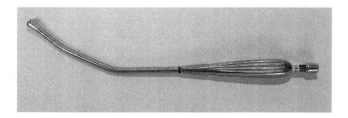

Yankauer Suction
(original photograph K. Roeder)

Sidney Yankauer (1872-1932) was a pioneer in bronchoscopy and practiced otolaryngology at Mt. Sinai Hospital in New York. He developed a tube suction device for the mouth and throat. His tonsil suction tip can be found in every operating room throughout the world in either a plastic or stainless steel version.

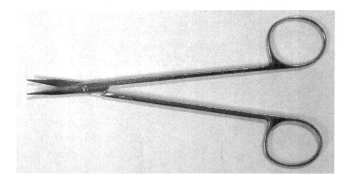

Stevens Scissors
(original photograph K. Roeder)

George Thomas Stevens (1833-1921), a Civil War surgeon, was a professor of physiology and diseases of the eye in New York. In 1889, he described his technique for correcting strabismus, using scissors he designed.

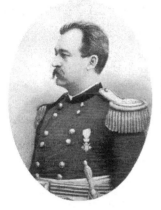

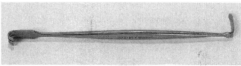

Senn Retractor
(original photograph K. Roeder)

Nicholas Senn
(Public Domain National Library of Medicine)

Nicholas Senn (1844-1908) was a Swiss born graduate of the Chicago Medical School who became Professor of Surgery at Rush Medical College. He was the first editor in chief of *Surgery, Gynecology and Obstetrics (SG&O)*, founder of the Military Association of Surgeons, and president of The American Medical Association. His retractor is typically used in operations on the hand and foot.

"The aim is to operate only when necessary but not to delay a necessary operation."

Moshe Schein

27

The Father of Surgical Education: William Halstead

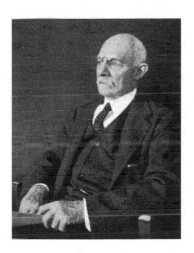

William Stewart Halsted
(Public Domain National Library of Medicine)

W illiam Stewart Halsted (September 23, 1852-September 7, 1922) was born in New York City the son of a wealthy textile importer. He entered Yale College in 1870 and was captain of the first Yale football team. After graduating from Yale he went to Columbia University College of Physicians and Surgeons in New York City. After graduating near the top of his medical school class, Halsted became a house physician at the New York Hospital. Like so many others of the day, Halsted travelled to Europe to observe and learn from famous European surgeons such as Chiari, Zuckerkandl, and Billroth. He studied their surgical techniques, research, and their training programs. He returned to New York and operated at Roosevelt Hospital, the College of Physicians and Surgeons, Charity Hospital, and Bellevue Hospital. He was the only surgeon in New York at that time practicing Listerian antisepsis and Germanic aseptic technique. His fame grew as one of the best surgeons and teachers of the day. In 1884, Halsted became aware of a report extolling the local anesthetic properties of cocaine. He and a few of his colleagues began to experiment with the substance by using it on themselves and subsequently became addicted. During a hospitalization to cure his addiction to cocaine he became addicted to morphine. He remained addicted to both drugs for this rest of his life.

His friend William Welch at Johns Hopkins invited Halsted to join him in Baltimore and become the first Professor and Chief of the Department of Surgery at Johns Hopkins Hospital when it opened in May 1889. Halsted started the first formal surgical residency-training program in the United States. His training program was meant to teach the teachers of surgery. Of his seventeen residents, eleven went on to develop surgical training programs at universities throughout the United States.

Halsted was known for his strict attention to hemostasis (control of surgical bleeding), gentle handling of tissues, and meticulous anatomical dissection. His slow, methodical technique and obsessive record keeping became legendary. Even today these attributes are referred to as Halstedian technique by current professors of surgery. He also was among the first to scientifically investigate wound healing. It is said that Halsted brought laboratory science to the practice of surgery.

He developed a technique to surgically treat the advanced cases of breast cancer seen routinely in his time and the technique became widely known as the Halsted mastectomy, which became the standard of treatment for 90 years.

At age 70, he was operated on for gallbladder disease and developed complications. He died on September 7, 1922. He is buried in Greenwood Cemetery in Brooklyn, New York. His wife Caroline, for whom he had the first rubber surgical gloves made, died just four months later.

"The only weapon with which the unconscious patient can immediately retaliate upon the incompetent surgeon is hemorrhage."

William Halstead

28

The Father of Modern Hernia Surgery: Eduardo Bassini

The standard hernia repair from the 1880s until the 1980s was the the Bassini hernia repair. Edoardo Basssini (April 14, 1844-July 19, 1924) reported the results of 206 hernia repairs using his method in 1884. He had an almost 100% five-year follow up rate for the 206 patients. The hernia recurrence rate at five years in those patients was slightly less than 4% and this was at a time when the recurrence rate was routinely much higher.

Bassini was born in Pavia, Italy. At the age of 22 he received his medical degree from the University of Pavia. He then joined the Italian Unification movement as an infantry soldier under Giuseppe Garibaldi during the Prussian-Austrian war. In 1867, he suffered a bayonet wound to the groin and was taken prisoner. Perhaps it was this wound that sparked his interest in groin anatomy. After the war, he studied in Vienna under Theodor Billroth and spent time with Bernhard von Langenbeck in Berlin, Germany. He travelled to London and studied with the likes of Joseph Lister. In 1882 he became head of surgical pathology at the University of Padua, and then appointed as chair of clinical surgery.

Bassini's operative technique for repair of inguinal hernia included suture reconstruction of the floor of the patients' inguinal canal after high ligation of the hernia sac. Bassini is also credited with the introduction of Listerian antiseptic practices into Italian surgery.

"Je le Pansai. Dieu le Guerit"
"I treated him. God cured him."

Ambrose Pare

29

The Father of Neurosurgery:
Harvey Cushing

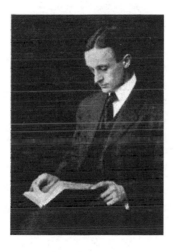

Harvey Williams Cushing
(Public Domain Copyright expired)

Harvey Williams Cushing (1869-1939) is considered to be the founding father of the specialty of neurosurgery. He was also a Pulitzer Prize winning author, medical historian, and an artist. He was born in Cleveland, Ohio in a long line of family physicians. He was the last of ten children. He graduated from Yale College and then from Harvard Medical School. He completed his internship at the Massachusetts General Hospital. He did his surgical training under William Halstead at the Johns

Hopkins Hospital but became close to William Osler, the Chief of Medicine, who became his mentor. He spent a year in Europe and trained with the great Theodor Kocher. He brought back the practice of intraoperative measurement of blood pressure to North America. He played a major role in the development of the electrocautery along with physicist W.T. Bovie.

He experimented on the function of the pituitary gland in the animal model and developed techniques and instruments to operate on tumors of the pituitary.

Harvey Cushing's name became forever associated with the disorders of the pituitary gland. Cushing's Disease refers to a pituitary-dependent cause of Cushing's syndrome: a tumor (adenoma) in the pituitary gland produces large amounts of adrenocorticotrophic hormone (ACTH) causing the adrenal glands to produce elevated levels of cortisol. He wrote a biography of Sir William Osler and became the only surgeon to ever win the famed Pulitzer Prize for literature. He died of a heart attack in 1939 and is buried in Lakeview Cemetery in Cleveland, Ohio.

"I would like to see the day when somebody would be appointed surgeon somewhere who had no hands, for the operative part is the least part of the work."

Harvey Cushing

30

The Father of Pediatric Surgery: William Ladd

William Edwards Ladd, M.D. (1880-1967) was born into an affluent New England family in 1880. He attended private preparatory schools, graduated from Harvard, and received his M.D. from Harvard Medical School in 1906. He completed his residency in general surgery at Boston City Hospital.

In 1917, a French cargo ship loaded with wartime explosives hit a Norwegian ship in Halifax harbor. The resulting explosion left over 2,000 dead and approximately 9,000 injured. Dr. Ladd was part of a medical team sent by express train to treat the injured. Ladd treated hundreds of burned and injured children during this tragedy and as a result, when he returned, limited his practice to the surgery of infants and children. He was named Chief of Surgery of the Boston Children's Hospital in 1927. He was the first to develop a training program in pediatric surgery.

Ladd preached that infants and children are not small adults and should be cared for by those who devote their talents to the treatment of infants and children only. He wrote the book on pediatric surgery when he co-authored with Robert Gross the first textbook on pediatric surgery entitled *Abdominal Surgery of Infancy and Childhood.*

His accomplishments and innovations in pediatric surgery are innumerable. His research and work led to a change and/or improvement in the treatment of tracheoesophageal fistula, extrophy of the bladder, the surgery of Wilm's Tumor, intussusception, and pyloric stenosis.

He is best known for the Ladd's Procedure he developed for the treatment of midgut volvulus. He emphasized the importance of dividing the congenital bands over the duodenum, placing the caecum in the left upper quadrant, and performing an appendectomy. He died at the age of 87 in Boston. He was the undisputed father of pediatric surgery.

"To study medicine without books is to sail an uncharted sea, while to study medicine only from books is not to go to sea at all."

Sir William Osler

31

The Father of Modern Orthopedics: Willis Campbell

Willis C. Campbell (1880-1941) was born in Jackson, Mississippi in 1880 and graduated from University of Virginia College of Medicine in 1904. After his internship, Dr. Campbell began his practice in Memphis, specializing in general surgery, anesthesia, and pediatrics. He travelled to Europe to study orthopedics in London and Vienna. When he returned to Memphis, Tennessee in 1909 he began his practice of orthopedic surgery.

In 1910, Dr. Campbell organized the Department of Orthopedic Surgery at the newly developed University of Tennessee in Memphis and became the first professor and head of that department. By 1924, he had begun the first orthopedic residency training program at UT Memphis. In 1933, he founded the American Academy of Orthopedic Surgeons and became its first president. He published his famous textbook *Campbell's Operative Orthopedics* in 1939. This text, now in its 11th edition, is used the world over and is the Bible of orthopedic surgery.

"The greater the ignorance the greater the dogmatism."
Sir William Osler

32

The Father of Cardiac Surgery: Michael DeBakey

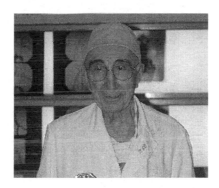

Michael Ellis DeBakey
(Public Domain US NASA)

Michael Ellis Debakey (September 7, 1908-July 12, 2008) was born in Lake Charles, Louisiana. He received his Bachelor of Science degree from Tulane University and his M.D. from Tulane University School of Medicine. He remained in New Orleans to complete his surgical residency training at the famed Charity Hospital. In 1939, while at Tulane along with his friend and mentor, Alton Ochsner, he proposed the link between smoking and lung cancer. DeBakey travelled to Europe to complete a surgical fellowship with Leriche at the University of Strasbourg in France and then studied at the University of Heidelberg, Germany under Professor Martin

Kirschner. He came back to Tulane and was on the surgical staff there until 1942.

During World War II, he joined the Surgical Consultants' Division in the Office of the Surgeon General of the Army. He helped change the care of the wounded soldier by developing aide stations near the front lines. This concept would lead to the mobile army surgical hospital or MASH units in the Korean War. Upon his return from the army, he joined the surgical faculty of Baylor University College of Medicine in 1948. He served as the Chairman of the Department of Surgery there until 1993. He was also the Olga Keith Wiess and Distinguished Service Professor in the Michael E. DeBakey Department of Surgery at Baylor College of Medicine and Director of the DeBakey Heart Center for Research and Public Education at Baylor College of Medicine and the Methodist Hospital.

Dr. DeBakey was among the first to do coronary artery bypass surgery, the first to perform a successful carotid endarterectomy, and the first to use an external heart pump successfully in a human. He developed and championed the use of Dacron grafts to bypass or replace narrowed or blocked arteries. Working with Dr. Robert Jarvik, he helped develop the first artificial heart.

DeBakey received many prestigious honors and awards for his work. These include the Presidential Medal of Freedom, the United Nations Lifetime Achievement Award, and the Congressional Gold Medal, among many others.

At age 98 he underwent surgery to repair a torn aorta, which was a procedure he had developed some fifty years earlier. Dr. Michael DeBakey lived another two years and died in Houston, Texas of natural causes just before his 100th birthday. He is buried in Arlington National Cemetery.

"Young surgeons err in believing that knowledge can compensate for lack of experience: old surgeons err in believing that experience can compensate for lack of knowledge."
Anonymous

33

The Father of Modern Gynecology: J. Marion Simms

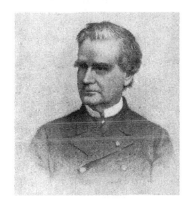

J. Marion Simms

J. Marion Simms was born in Hanging Rock, South Carolina. He graduated from Jefferson Medical College in Philadelphia, Pennsylvania in 1835. He then moved to Montgomery, Alabama. A pioneer in vaginal surgery, Dr. Sims developed a surgical treatment for vesicovaginal fistulas (a complication of childbirth in which abnormal connections develop between a woman's bladder and vagina, leading to incontinence and unpleasantness). Unfortunately Simms did this by experimenting on black women, who at the time were slaves. He unforgivably operated without anesthesia and in some individuals did more than thirty procedures while perfecting his technique.

Sims invented his own instruments, including the speculum used for exposure of the vagina and cervix that bears his name. His use of silver-wire sutures led to the successful repair of a vesicovaginal fistula, which he published in 1852.

Sims founded the first hospital for women in America in New York City. He left the United States during the Civil War and travelled to Europe, residing and practicing mainly in London and Paris.

In 1871, Sims returned to New York and became the President of the American Medical Association in 1876. Because of his work, gynecology became recognized as a separate specialty and he is hailed as its father. A statue of him can be found in Central Park across from the Academy of Medicine. He died at the age of 70 of heart failure and is buried in Brooklyn, New York.

"It is astonishing with how little reading a doctor can practice medicine, but it is not astonishing how badly he may do it."
Sir William Osler

34

The Blue Baby Turns Pink

The anesthesiologist excitedly told the surgeon to look at the difference in the color of the nine-pound fifteen month-old baby girl lying on the operating room table. In the moments before the arterial shunt was connected, little Eileen had a mottled blue color. Now she was pink and appeared healthy. When the surgeon, Alfred Blalock, peered over the drapes at the head of the operating room table, he must have known at that moment that a real advance in heart surgery had finally been realized. He had come a long way to get to that moment.

In 1899, Alfred Blalock was born just west of Macon, Georgia in the small town of Culloden. After graduating from the University of Georgia, he moved to Baltimore, Maryland and completed his medical degree at Johns Hopkins University. After three years of unsuccessfully trying to obtain a residency at Johns Hopkins, he moved to Vanderbilt University Hospital in Nashville to become the first resident in surgery there. It was here that Blalock discovered that the cause of traumatic shock was the loss of blood and advocated the use of plasma and whole blood in the treatment of shock. This discovery saved the lives of countless soldiers during the Second World War.

In 1941 Blalock returned to Johns Hopkins to become a professor and Director of the Department of Surgery. Luckily he took Vivian Thomas, his laboratory assistant, with him. Thomas was a talented and brilliant African-American, and Blalock had refused to go without him.

At Johns Hopkins, Blalock and Thomas continued their work with the development of a technique of shunting blood around a constriction in the main artery leaving the heart, a condition called coarctation of the aorta. Their method involved dividing and using the subclavian artery as a conduit. Helen Taussig, the mother of pediatric cardiology, suggested that perhaps the shunt could be utilized in children with blue baby syndrome—Tetralogy of Fallot. This congenital heart defect results in blood with poor oxygenation being delivered to the body. The poor oxygenation results from the fact that the outflow tract from the right ventricle to the pulmonary artery is constricted and blood flow is impeded. Also, there is a hole in the septum between the right and left ventricles. This septal defect allows the higher-pressure oxygenated blood to be shunted through the defect into the right ventricle and therefore not to the body.

Dr. Taussig thought the same type of shunt could alleviate the problem. Thomas and Blalock developed the technique of dividing the subclavian artery and turning it down to connect to the pulmonary artery. This took a large amount of the poorly oxygenated blood and put it back through the pulmonary circulation. After many animal experiments, on November 29, 1944 with Taussig looking on and Thomas standing behind him, Blalock, assisted by his resident William Longmire, M.D., performed the first Blalock-Taussig shunt for Tetralogy of Fallot. Blalock and Taussig published the results of three successful shunt operations in the *Journal of the American Medical Association* in May of 1945. This publication brought many blue babies from all over the world to Johns Hopkins and by 1952 more than a thousand such operations had been performed. In 2004, the movie "Something the Lord Made," recounting this inspiring story, was released.

Blalock was recognized with many honors and awards including a clinical science building named after him at Johns

Hopkins. Vivian Thomas was awarded an honorary degree of Doctor of Laws, also at Johns Hopkins. His portrait hangs next to Blalock's at the Alfred Blalock Clinical Sciences Building on the campus of Johns Hopkins Hospital.

"Science is the father of knowledge, but opinion breeds ignorance."

Hippocrates of Cos

35

John H. Gibbon:
The Birth of Open-Heart Surgery

B efore 1953, open-heart surgery was only a dream. In 1923, at the Peter Bent Brigham Hospital in Boston, a successful case of a closed mitral valve commissurotomy opened the door to successfully operating on the heart. However, intracardiac surgery required a method to divert the blood flow away from the heart and lungs so that the surgeon could work. The birth of open-heart surgery awaited Dr. John H. Gibbon's invention of a pump oxygenator.

John Heysham Gibbon was born in Philadelphia, Pennsylvania 1903. He was a fourth generation physician. He graduated from Princeton University and then received his medical degree from Jefferson Medical College in Philadelphia in 1927. In 1930, he obtained a research fellowship with Dr. Edward Churchill, the famous chief of surgery at the Massachusetts General Hospital in Boston.

On October 3, 1930, Dr. Gibbon witnessed the collapse of a patient as a result of a massive pulmonary embolism occurring two weeks after a gallbladder operation. After a period of deteriorating blood pressure and vital signs, witnessed by Gibbon who stayed at the patient's bedside all night, Dr. Churchill opened the patient's chest. He then opened the pulmonary artery, removed the clot, and closed the pulmonary artery (Trendelenburg operation)—all in six minutes. As was usual for this operation, the patient died.

This experience had a tremendous effect on Gibbon and set the course of the rest of his life.

Gibbon approached Churchill with the idea that perhaps a machine could take over the oxygenation of the blood if the pulmonary artery became obstructed. Churchill reluctantly agreed to keep him on for another year of fellowship to research the idea. Gibbon knew the four main components that such a machine would need would be a venous reservoir, an oxygenator, a temperature regulator for the extracorporeal blood, and an arterial pump. He set about developing the machine and finding the appropriate materials.

After an initial design, which actually kept a cat alive for twenty-six minutes, Gibbon had to stop his efforts when he was called to serve in the army during World War II. On his return from the war, he became Professor of Surgery at Jefferson and resumed his research. He met and began a collaboration with Thomas Watson. Watson, an engineer and the chairman of IBM (International Business Machines), provided the financial and technical support for Gibbon to further develop his heart-lung machine. A new device was developed that used a refined method that made the blood flow down a thin sheet of film allowing for oxygenation, rather than the original whirling technique that could potentially damage blood cells. Gibbon and IBM engineers had invented an improved machine that "minimized hemolysis and prevented air bubbles from entering the circulation."

The device was only tested on dogs and had a 10% mortality rate. After one failed attempt in humans, Gibbon tried again on May 6, 1953. The patient was an eighteen year-old girl, Cecelia Bavolek, who had been admitted several times with congestive heart failure due to an atrial septal defect (a hole in the septum between the upper chambers of the heart that allowed high pressure blood from the left side to flow into the right heart causing right heart failure). After full heparinization her heart was stopped and she was placed on full cardiac bypass for 26 minutes while Gibbon closed the septal defect with a running cotton suture. She was sent home thirteen days after surgery and had an uneventful recovery. She underwent re-catheterization six months after the procedure, and the defect remained completely closed. The world had witnessed the first open-heart operation and the dream of centuries became a reality for millions to follow.

Dr. Gibbon soon gave up cardiac surgery and returned to general thoracic surgery. He became Professor and Chairman of Surgery at Jefferson and was the President of the American Surgical Association in 1954 and the American Association of Thoracic Surgery in 1961. His many other awards included an honorary fellowship in the Royal College of Surgeons. He died in 1973 at age 69 of a fatal heart attack while playing tennis.

"Experience is the best teacher. Unfortunately experience causes mental scars and scar tissue contracts."

William Mayo

36

A Button and the Surgical Clinics of North America

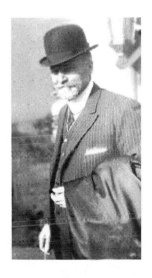

John Benjamin Murphy
(Public Domain Copyright Expired)

John Benjamin Murphy (1857-1916) was born December 21, 1857 in Appleton, Wisconsin. He was an American physician and abdominal surgeon noted for advocating early surgical intervention in appendicitis. He is best remembered for the Murphy's Sign, a clinical sign (tenderness in the right upper quadrant of the abdomen during inspiration) that is used in the examination of patients with possible acute inflammation of the gallbladder. He was indeed the true general surgeon as his practice and interests included general surgery, neurosurgery, and cardiothoracic surgery. Dr. William Mayo described him as "the surgical genius of our generation." He performed and developed innovative techniques in essentially every subspecialty of surgery.

Murphy attended public school in Appleton and then obtained a doctorate from Rush Medical College in 1879. He completed an internship at Cook County Hospital in Chicago he then travelled to Europe and worked at universities and hospitals in Vienna, Munich, Berlin and Heidelberg. Most of this time was spent working in Vienna with the great Theodor Billroth.

Murphy held positions at Rush Medical College, the College of Physicians and Surgeons, and at Northwestern University Medical School. He also taught at the Graduate Medical School of Chicago, and was the surgeon-in-chief at the Mercy Hospital until his death in 1916.

While at Mercy, he developed his wet clinics, in which he would simultaneously operate and lecture to an audience. Physicians from throughout the United States, as well as Europe and Asia, would come to watch and learn from Dr. Murphy. During these demonstrations, his teachings would be transcribed and they were printed as *The Surgical Clinics of John B. Murphy, M.D., at Mercy Hospital, Chicago,* which later became *The Surgical Clinics of Chicago,* and then, *Surgical Clinics of North America,* which is still in publication today.

He was considered pretentious by many of his professional colleagues in the U.S. He advocated early appendectomy in all cases of appendicitis. This approach was controversial at that time when conservative management of appendicitis was the accepted treatment. Notwithstanding his unpopularity among his peers, he was eventually elected president of both the Chicago Medical Society and the American Medical Association (AMA).

He invented a button to perform intestinal anastomoses. The Murphy button can be credited as the forerunner of the modern end-to-end stapling instrument after having become the method of choice for operations at the Mayo Clinic and elsewhere in the United States for over twenty years.

"It usually requires a considerable time to determine with certainty the virtues of a new method of treatment and usually still longer to ascertain the harmful effects."

Alfred Blalock

37

Surgeon Nobel Laureates

There have been nine surgeons who have been awarded the Nobel Prize in Physiology and Medicine. In chronological order they are as follows: **Theodor Kocher in** 1909 for his advances in thyroid surgery and physiology of the thyroid gland; **Allvar Gullstrand** in 1911 for his work on the optics of the eye; **Alexis Carrel** in 1912 for his technique of vascular suturing and organ transplantation; **Robert Barany** for his work on the vestibular system (He was notified of his prize while in a Russian prisoner of war camp in 1914); **Frederick Banting** in 1923, for the discovery of insulin; **Walter Hess** in 1949 for the mapping and description of midbrain function; **Werner Forssmann** in 1956 for discovering the technique of cardiac catheterization; **Charles Huggins** in 1966 for his work with hormonal treatment of prostatic cancer; and **Joseph Murray**, in 1990 for his work with organ transplantation.

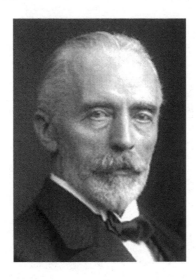

Emil Theodor Kocher

(Public Domain National Institutes of Health)

Emil Theodor Kocher was born in Berne, Switzerland in 1841. He completed medical school in Berne and then traveled and studied with Lister and Billroth. He returned to Berne and his clinic utilized Listerian antiseptic techniques. He has many contributions to surgery and but he received the 1909 Nobel Prize for his writings and work on the physiology, pathology, and surgical treatment of disorders of the thyroid gland.

In the late 1800s surgical procedures on the thyroid carried a high mortality rate. Iodine deficiency can result in goiter and in many areas around the world where the soil is deficient in iodine, the chemical must be added to the diet in the form of iodized salt. Before this was known, extremely large goiters were commonplace. Kocher's technique of ligation of both thyroid arteries prior to his precise anatomical dissection markedly reduced the blood loss leading to a lower mortality rate. Kocher noted that great care must be taken to avoid the recurrent laryngeal nerve to prevent the vocal changes and hoarseness that was so common following thyroid surgery. He developed partial thyroidectomy after seeing patients return with myxedema or hypothyroidism many years after total thyroidectomy. The Kocher clamp that he developed for hemostasis is used in every operating room in the world.

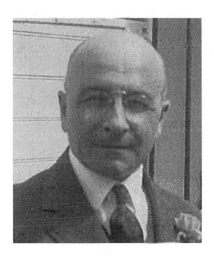

Alexis Carrel
(Public Domain Library of Congress)

Alexis Carrel was a French physician who worked in the United States, first at the University of Chicago and then at the Rockefeller Institute. Carrel received the Nobel Prize in Physiology or Medicine in 1912 for developing new methods for suturing small blood vessels. He had gone to the best embroiderer in Lyons and learned how to use very small needles and fine silk. Soon his technical skill was even better than his teachers. He perfected the triangulation method of vascular anastomosis.

In 1935, Carrel along with Charles Lindberg developed a perfusion pump that oxygenated living organs and kept them viable outside the body. This advance was a key element in the development of organ transplantation. He wrote a book with Lindbergh entitled *The Culture of Organs,* and they were featured on the cover of *Time* magazine in 1938.

Every surgeon has heard of Dakin's solution, and it was Carrel and English chemist Henry Dakin who developed the sodium hypochlorite solution used as a wound antiseptic in World War I. Because of his work Carrel was hailed as a national hero in France; however, a few years prior he had written a book *Man, the Unknown*, in which he advocated eugenics. He stated that man could control his destiny by allowing only the strong and biologically worthwhile to be perpetuated. At that same time, Hitler's Nazi Germany was advocating eugenics and Nazi leaders endorsed Carrel's work. After the war his public image went from scientific hero to hated Nazi sympathizer. It has been said that he died of sorrow because of the negative opinion that people came to have of him.

Joseph Murray

Joseph Murray was awarded the prize in 1990 for his groundbreaking efforts in the field of organ transplantation. He was born in 1919 and attended Harvard Medical School and graduated in 1943. He then spent three years in the U.S. Army and following his discharge completed a surgical residency and a fellowship in plastic and reconstructive surgery at Harvard.

Others had attempted kidney transplantation using cadaver kidneys without success due to immunological rejection. Also, the transplanted kidneys were placed in the recipients' thighs. Richard Herrick, a 24 year-old man dying of kidney failure, presented for treatment to the Peter Bent Brigham Hospital in Boston. The patient underwent kidney dialysis. His twin brother's skin was grafted onto him and there was complete take of the graft, which confirmed they were identical.

Murray had auto-transplanted kidneys in dogs and utilized the abdominal cavity as the site of transplantation. On December 23, 1954, Richard Herrick was taken to the operating room and Dr. Murray transplanted the normal kidney of his identical twin brother Ronald into the dying Richard. The postoperative course was completely successful, and the patient left the hospital within a few weeks. The first successful organ transplant had occurred, and a new era of surgery had begun.

Murray would transplant two fraternal twins in 1959 following whole body irradiation for immunosuppression. Then in 1962 he utilized drugs to obtain immunosuppression and this became the model for all future organ transplants.

"The incision should always be as long as is needed and as short as possible."

Emil Theodor Kocher

38

Electrosurgery and a Man Named Bovie

Electrosurgery is the passing of a high-frequency alternating current into the body as a means to cut or coagulate tissue. Heat has been used for surgical procedures for thousands of years. A hot iron or fire stick was used to treat tumors and ulcers of all types in ancient Egypt. Hippocrates treated hemorrhoids with cauterization. It was common practice to treat war wounds and amputations with boiling oil up until the middle of the 16th century.

In the early 1900's Dr. Simon Pozi used high voltage low amperage current to treat cancers of the skin. He named the technique fulguration. Using a grounding plate that allowed deeper tissue penetration, Eugene Doyen coined the term electrocoagulation. In 1910, Dr. William Clark of Philadelphia increased the amperage, decreased the voltage, and utilized multiple spark gaps instead of the commonly used single gap. Under the microscope he noticed that his technique caused the tissue to shrink and he coined the term desiccation.

William T. Bovie had a master's degree in botany and a doctorate in plant physiology from Harvard University. Bovie's device used a high frequency current delivered by a cutting loop that could cut, coagulate, or desiccate.

Surgeons were slow to use the device until 1926 when the famous neurosurgeon Harvey Cushing expressed an interest. On October 1, 1926, Dr. Cushing used Bovie's electrosurgical unit to successfully remove a vascular myeloma from the head of a

64 year-old patient. Cushing and Bovie continued to improve the device and Bovie sold his patent rights for one dollar to the Liebel-Florshwim Company that made it widely available for use.

Bovie's electrocautery unit greatly enhances surgical technique by decreasing tissue damage, preventing blood loss, and decreasing operative time. His work has impacted millions of patients and although he died a poor man, generations of surgeons have called out his name every day in every operating room as they say, "Bovie please".

"A surgeon is a physician who can't wait to get into the operating room and, once there, can't wait to get out."

Jonathan R. Hiatt

39

Johns Hopkins and the Four Physicians

Johns Hopkins was born in 1795 on a tobacco plantation in Anne Arundel County, Maryland. His first name is after the last name of his great grandmother Margaret Johns. He was from a family of Quakers. At age 17 he left his home and moved to Baltimore to work in his uncle's wholesale grocery. There he fell in love with his cousin Elizabeth. Because of the Quaker prohibition against the marriage of first cousins, they never married. After seven years, he left his uncle's business and developed many businesses of his own with his brothers. The great majority of his wealth came from shrewd investments. Most of his fortune was from his investment in the Baltimore and Ohio Railroad. Before and during the Civil War, he was an abolitionist and a great supporter of Abraham Lincoln and the Union, which put him at odds with most Marylanders.

He died at age 78 on Christmas Eve in 1873. A bachelor with no children, he bequeathed the largest monetary gift in the history of the United States, the amazing sum of seven million dollars, to establish a university and a hospital in Baltimore, Maryland. Hopkins' instruction letter explicitly stated his vision for the hospital: first, to provide assistance to the poor of "all races"; second, that wealthier patients would pay for services and thereby subsidize the care provided to the indigent; third, that the hospital would be the administrative unit for the orphan asylum for African American children; and finally, that the hospital should be part of the university.

The university and the hospital opened in 1889. The medical school was to open at the same time, but the price of the B&O stock had fallen and there was a lack of $500,000 in order to open the medical school. A four-woman committee headed by Mary Elizabeth Garrett promised to raise the needed funds with the following provisos: 1) Women were to be admitted with the same basis as men. 2) The medical school had to be a graduate school. 3) The students were to have a broad undergraduate education and a high-grade average. The money was raised, and in 1893 the Johns Hopkins School of Medicine was opened. In his 1910 report on the state of medical education in America, Abraham Flexner used The Johns Hopkins School of Medicine as the ideal model of what U.S. medical schools should be.

William Henry Welch, M.D. became the first Professor and Chairman of the Department of Pathology. He trained many famous physicians including Walter Reed. He established the first school of public health in the U.S. He was also responsible in part for the recruitment of William Halstead and Sir William Osler.

William Halstead became the first Professor and Chairman of Surgery. He modeled his surgical training program after the German one of the day. He trained many future famous chairmen of departments of surgery. His story is detailed elsewhere in this book, but his work on surgical education, local anesthesia and subsequent cocaine addiction is well known. His name is known and routinely spoken by every modern day surgeon.

Sir William Osler became the first Professor and Chairman of the Department of Internal Medicine. He was known to be an excellent teacher and perhaps the most famous physician of the day. He believed in teaching at the bedside, and his quotes and aphorisms fill books. Osler brought Howard Kelly to the Johns Hopkins School of Medicine. Kelly became the first Professor and Chairman of the Department of Gynecology. Kelly concentrated on understanding the underlying pathology of women's diseases and invented many instruments including the cystoscope.

John Singer Sargent's famous 1907 portrait, *Four Physicians*, depicts Welch, Kelly, Halstead, and Osler surrounding a massive Venetian globe. The painting hangs in the Welch Medical Library at Johns Hopkins University. It was was commissioned and dedicated to Mary Elizabeth Garrett.

"Live neither in the past nor in the future, but let each day's work absorb your entire energies, and satisfy your widest ambition."

Sir William Osler, to his students

40

The Mayo Clinic and the Mayo Brothers

B rothers William and Charles Mayo, both surgeons, founded the famous Mayo Clinic in Rochester, Minnesota, one of the first efforts at multispecialty group practice in the United States. William was born in Le Sueur, Minnesota in 1861, and his brother Charles followed four years later in Rochester, Minnesota. They were the sons of William Worrall Mayo, a country doctor who settled in Minnesota after emigrating from England in 1845. They frequently traveled with their father on his house calls. Both chose medicine as a career. William graduated from the University of Michigan and then continued his training in New York. Charles went to the Chicago Medical School (later to be known as Northwestern). William was said to be quiet and reserved while his younger brother Charles was outgoing and friendly.

In 1883, a tornado struck Rochester, Minnesota and Dr. William Worrall Mayo and his two sons began treating the victims in a dance hall. They enlisted the help of Mother Alfred Moes and the Sisters of Saint Francis. Mother Alfred then began to raise money to build a hospital and involved the three Mayo doctors in the planning and staffing of the hospital. In 1889, the Sisters of Saint Francis opened the doors to St. Mary's Hospital in Rochester. There were twenty-seven beds. On September 30, 1889, Dr. Charles Mayo performed the first operation, and his brother assisted him as his father gave the anesthetic. The Mayos named their part of the hospital the Mayo Clinic. By 1900 over three thousand operations a year would take place. What began as a surgical clinic would become a medical center, a philanthropic foundation, and a graduate school of medicine.

The Mayo brothers took leave three months a year apiece at separate times and traveled and operated extensively with the experts in Europe and in America. Many physicians and surgeons came to visit them in Rochester. They attracted many leaders in surgery and medicine and convinced them to stay in Rochester. Both brothers would serve in the U.S. Army during World War I. They reached the rank of Brigadier General and received the Distinguished Service Medal. William went on to become the president of the American Medical Association and published more than six hundred scientific articles.

At the age of 88, their father, Dr. William Worrall Mayo, got his hand stuck in a machine he was attempting to repair and eventually the hand required amputation. After the accident his health declined steadily, and he died at the age of 92. Dr. Charles Mayo died of lobar pneumonia at the age of 73 in 1939. Two months later, his brother Dr. Will Mayo died in his sleep of a stomach malignancy.

Of course the Mayo Clinic is now a giant multi-institution system of health care with satellite facilities throughout the United States. But it was a tornado in Rochester that started the winds of change in private multispecialty health care in America.

"Each day as I go through the hospital surrounded by young men, they give me of their dreams and I give them of my experience. And, I get the better of the exchange."

William Mayo

ADDENDUM: PRESIDENTIAL PATIENTS

─────── I ───────

George Washington, President 1789-1797

One cold December morning in 1799, President Washington went horseback riding at his Mount Vernon estate. The next day he was hoarse and had a sore throat. The following night he told his wife Martha that he was experiencing severe throat pain and was having difficulty breathing. Dr. James Craik, Washington's personal physician, was called to see him. Dr. Craik examined Washington on the morning of Dec. 14, 1799, and made a diagnosis of "inflammatory quinsy" (Peritonsillar abscess) or epiglottitis. Craik declared the condition life threatening and quickly called together a team of doctors to care for the President. They all agreed that the cause of his illness was the larynx and they bled him of five pints of blood, burned his neck, and gave him purgatives. These practices sound outlandish but were the accepted medical treatments of the day. He died 12 hours later of his airway obstructing epiglottitis. He was 67 years old.

"The most common cause of postoperative coagulopathy: poor hemostasis. The most important clotting factor is the surgeon."

Anonymous

II

James A. Garfield, President 1881

Of the four American presidents who have been assassinated, James Garfield, the twentieth American president, was the second. In 1881, Charles Guiteau became interested in politics after failing in several other endeavors. He wrote and delivered a speech in support of Garfield's election. For this he felt he was due the ambassadorship to Paris. When the Garfield administration refused Guiteau's repeated requests, he bought a .44 caliber revolver, went to the Sixth Street train station and lay in wait for President Garfield. Garfield, just four months into his presidency, was about to leave for Massachusetts to deliver a speech. On July 2, 1881, with Robert Todd Lincoln standing near Garfield's side, Guiteau shot President James Garfield once through the arm and the second shot struck the President in the back.

The first doctor on the scene gave him spirits of ammonia and caused him to vomit. He was taken to the White House and a leading surgeon of the day, Dr. D.W. Bliss, took complete charge of the President's care. He stuck his unwashed ungloved finger into the wound and then an unclean metal probe was used. Many others probed the president's wound with unclean instruments searching for the bullet. For weeks Garfield suffered and could not eat. His weight went from 210 pounds to 130 pounds.

The famous Philadelphia surgeon David Hayes Agnew made an incision into the tract hoping to drain pus. Alexander Graham Bell invented a metal detector and tried to locate the bullet on two occasions. Because of the oppressive Washington summer heat, Garfield was moved by train to the New Jersey shore.

After two and a half months of suffering, Garfield died of overwhelming infection on September 19, 1881. Guiteau's attorneys argued that it was the surgeons who caused the death of the president by introducing infection into an otherwise non-fatal wound. In hindsight they were right. Charles Julius Guiteau was found guilty of murder and executed by hanging on June 30, 1882 at the age of forty-two.

"If a surgeon is asked to name the three best surgeons in town, he is hard pressed to name the other two."

Anonymous

III

Grover Cleveland, President 1885-1889, 1893-1897

The *Oneida* was a 138-foot luxury yacht owned by Elias Benedict who was a close friend of President Cleveland, our 22nd and 24th President. On July 1, 1893, as the *Oneida* made its way up Long Island Sound with Cleveland on board, the President was undergoing a secret operation. He had noticed an enlarging lump on the roof of his mouth but had ignored it due to a growing financial crisis in the country. The railroads were overbuilt and going bankrupt and with that came the possibility of a stock market failure and rising unemployment. Also, the nation debated over whether the dollar should be backed by gold or silver. When President Cleveland finally asked his personal physician, Dr. Joseph Bryant, to examine the growth, Bryant advised immediate removal. Cleveland did not want the public to know about his surgery, fearing that knowledge of his incapacity could increase the country's financial instability. A surgical team of experts headed by Dr. Bryant was assembled and all the necessary equipment was placed on board the yacht.

Bryant, assisted by a dentist and three other doctors, including W.W. Keen of Philadelphia, removed the cancerous tumor while Cleveland sat in a chair in the yacht's main stateroom. Five days later he was dropped off at his summer home in Massachusetts as if nothing had happened. He was fitted with a rubber plate for the roof of his mouth and his speaking voice was then normal. The story broke in a Philadelphia newspaper the following month, but

Cleveland flatly denied the event and no one believed the story. The facts never came out until Keen published an account of the operation in 1917 in the *Saturday Evening Post*, some eight years after President Cleveland's death.

"The lowest mortality and fewest complications result from the removal of normal tissue."

Mark Ravitch

IV

Dwight Eisenhower, President 1953-1961

D wight Eisenhower developed vague, ill-defined discomfort in the lower abdomen at 12:30 a.m. on June 8, 1956. His physician arrived at the White House thirty minutes later and found the President to have a moderately distended abdomen, but with no particular point of abdominal tenderness. He was given tap water enemas with no relief, and he then began to vomit. When seen by a consultant, Eisenhower was listless, apathetic, and perspiring freely. He had somewhat cool and clammy skin and a pulse of 120. The President was transferred to Walter Reed General Hospital.

By 1:00 a.m. on June 9, the distention of the small bowel, seen on the initial X-ray, was increasing. Consulting surgeons unanimously felt surgical intervention was indicated. At 2:20 a.m. the President's operation began. At operation, the last foot and a half of the small intestine had the typical appearance of chronic regional enteritis (Crohn's Disease). The obstructed segment was bypassed. The procedure went smoothly and one pint of blood was transfused.

Eisenhower's post-operative course was uneventful save for a fever and minor wound infection. He began conducting official business of the Presidency on the fifth day after the operation.

"Reprimand the surgery resident who errs and fire the one who lies."

Anonymous

V

Ronald Reagan, President 1981-1989

The movie *Taxi Driver* starring Robert De Niro and Jodie Foster released in 1976. The story was loosely based on the life of Arthur Bremmer, a loner who was enamored of and rejected by his girlfriend. He then shaved his head, starting acting strangely, and in order to prove his manhood, decided to assassinate President Richard Nixon. However, because of the tight security surrounding the President, Bremmer instead decided to kill the Democratic candidate for President of the United States, Governor George Wallace. On May 15, 1972 he shot and paralyzed George Wallace in a shopping center parking lot in Laurel, Maryland.

John Hinckley, Jr. saw the movie *Taxi Driver* fifteen times and became obsessed with the actress Jodie Foster. He stalked her, called her, and enrolled in a course at Yale University just to be near her. She refused to meet with him or return his calls. In order to gain Ms. Foster's attention, Hinckley decided to assassinate President Ronald Reagan, who had defeated Jimmy Carter in the 1980 Presidential election and on January 20, 1981 became the 40th President of the United States.

On March 30, 1981 at 2:27 p.m. outside the Washington Hilton Hotel, 26 year-old John Hinckley, Jr. fired his .22 caliber revolver at Reagan six times in less than two seconds. White House Press Secretary James Brady was struck in the head. A Washington, D.C. police officer, Thomas Delahanty was hit in the neck, and secret service agent Timothy McCarthy was shot in the abdomen. Reagan was pushed into the waiting limousine and it was later discovered that he had been shot in the chest.

Regan was taken to George Washington University Hospital. He collapsed as he walked through the emergency department door. His systolic blood pressure was 60 mmHg. Intravenous fluids raised his pressure to normal and E.D. physician Joseph Giordano placed a chest tube. Over two liters of blood came from the President's chest. An arterial line was placed and he was taken to operating room 2 at 2:57 p.m., just thirty minutes from the time of the shooting. A peritoneal lavage was negative for blood in the abdomen. Just before induction of anesthesia, Reagan said, "I hope you are all Republicans."

Dr. Benjamin Aaron performed a left thoracotomy to stop the lung from bleeding and remove the exploding bullet lodged within it. Reagan left the hospital seventeen days later. Hinckley was found not guilty by reason of insanity and is confined, except for controlled visits to his parents, at St. Elizabeth's Hospital in Washington D.C. He wrote that the shooting of President Reagan was "the greatest love offering in the history of the world."

"The art of medicine is to entertain the patient while nature cures the disease."

Voltaire

REFERENCES

Books:

- *Bulfinch's Mythology* (Modern Library Classics); Modern Library Reprint edition (August 11, 1998)
- Ellis, Harold: *A History of Surgery.* Greenwich Medical Media Limited. *London, England 2001.*
- Ellis, Harold: *Operations that Made History* (New York: Cambridge University Press, 1996)
- Ellis, Joseph J, *His Excellency, George Washington.* Vintage Books a division of Random House, New York, New York (2004)
- Hollingham, Richard: *Blood and Guts, A History of Surgery* New York: Thomas Dunne Books, St. Martin's Press (2008)
- Millard, Candice: *Destiny of the Republic: A Tale of Madness Medicine and the Murder of a President.* Anchor; Reprint edition (June 12, 2012)
- Nuland, Sherwin: *Doctors: The Biography of Medicine* (New York: Knopf, 1988
- Nuland, Sherwin: *Medicine: The Art of Healing* (New York: Hugh Lauter Levin Associates, Inc.: Distributed by Macmillan, 1992)
- Rutkow, Ira: *Surgery: An Illustrated History Mosby-Year Book (October 1, 1993)*
- Rutkow, Ira: American Surgery: An Illustrated History. Lippincott Williams & Wilkins; 1 Ed edition (January 15, 1998)

- Schwartz, Seymour: *Gifted Hands: America's Most Significant Contributions to Surgery*. Amherst, New York—Prometheus Books 2009
- Schein, Moshe. *Aphorisms and Quotations for the Surgeon*. Shrewsbury, UK. TFM Publishing, Ltd. 2004.
- Tilney, Nicholas: *Invasion of the Body* (Cambridge, Massachusetts, Harvard University Press, 2011)
- Wilber, Del Quetin: *Rawhide Down: The Near Assassination of Ronald Reagan* Henry Holt and Co.; First Edition (March 15, 2011)

Periodical Literature

- Cushing, HC: Electro-surgery as an aid to the removal of intracranial tumors. With a preliminary note on a new surgical current generator by W.T. Bovie, Ph.D. *Surg Gynecol Obstet 47: 751,1928*
- Sparkman, R.S.: The Woman in the Case. Jane Todd Crawford 1763-1842. *Ann Surg189: 529,1979*
- Long, C. W. (1849). An account of the first use of Sulphuric Ether by Inhalation as an Anaesthetic in Surgical Operations, *Southern Medical and Surgical Journal*, 5, 705-713
- Bears, OH. The medical history of President Ronald Reagan. *Surgery, Obstetrics, and Gynecology* 178:86-96, 1994
- Rutkow, I.M. A history of the Surgical Clinics of North America. *Surgical Clinics of North America* 67:1217-1239, 1987
- Kazi, RA; Peter, RE (2004). "Christian Albert Theodor Billroth: Master of surgery". *Journal of postgraduate medicine* 50 (1): 82-3. PMID 15048012.
- McBurney, Charles "Experience with Early Operative Interference in Cases of Disease of the Vermiform Appendix"; *New York Medical Journal*, 1889, 50: 676-684 [pg. 678].
- Whipple, A.O. "The surgical therapy of hyperinsulinism", in *J Internat Chir* 3:237-276 (1938)

- Bradley, Diana. Dr. Gibbon's heart-lung machine thrives against the odds. DOTmedbusiness news Sept 2012 pg. 73
- Caroline Hampton Halsted: the first to use rubber gloves in the operating room. Lathan R.S., MD Proc (Bayl Univ Med Cent). 2010 October; 23(4): 389-392.
- Blumhagen DW. The doctor's white coat: the image of the physician in modern America. *Ann Intern Med.* 1979;91:111-116.
- *Hochberg, MS, MD* The Doctor's White Coat—an Historical Perspective *Virtual Mentor.* April 2007, Volume 9, Number 4: 310-314.
- Laufman, H MD, PhD, Belkin, N PhD, Meyer, K, MD (FACS) A critical review of a century's progress in surgical apparel: how far have we come? Journal of the American College of Surgeons Vol. 191 issue 5, Pages 554-568, November 2000
- Ochsner, J. MD Surgical Knife Tex Heart Inst J. 2009; 36(5): 441-443.
- DeVoe, A.J. Ramon Castroviejo Trans Am Ophthalmol Soc. 1987; 85: 6-8.
- Duane, A. Stevens, G.T., M.D., Ph.D Trans Am Ophthalmol Soc. 1921:19: 14.2-19
- Nicholas Senn Club Dinner 1906.www.facs.org/archives/sennclubdinner.html
- Clifton G. Meals, BA, Roy A. Meals, MD (2007). "A History of Surgery in the Instrument Tray: Eponymous Tools Used in Hand Surgery". *Journal of Hand Surgery* 32 (7): 942-953.
- Cameron, John. (1997). "Williams Stewart Halsted: Our Surgical Heritage". *Annals of Surgery* 225 (5): 445-58.
- Bill H. William E. Ladd, M.D.: great pioneer of North American pediatric surgery. Prog Pediatr Surg. 1986; 20:52-9.
- Wall, LL. The medical ethics of Dr. J Marion Sims: a fresh look at the historical record Med Ethics. 2006 June; 32(6): 346-350
- Toledo-Pereyra, LH. Alfred Blalock. Surgeon, educator, and pioneer in shock and cardiac research. J Invest Surg. 2005 Jul-Aug; 18(4): 161-5

- *Blalock. A, Taussig, HB. The Surgical Treatment of Malformations of the Heart in Which There is Pulmonary Stenosis or Pulmonary Atresia. The Journal of the American Medical Association (128:189, May 19, 1945)*
- Fou, A.A. John H. Gibbon. The first 20 years of the heart-lung machine. Tex Heart Inst. J. 1997; 24(1): 1-8.
- Cutler EC, Levine SA. Cardiotomy and valvulotomy for mitral stenosis: experimental observations and clinical notes concerning an operated case with recovery. Boston Med Surg J. 1923; 188: 1023-1027.
- Gibbon JH Jr. Application of a mechanical heart and lung apparatus to cardiac surgery. Minn Med. 1954; 37: 171-180.
- Levison. CGT, he Surgical Clinics of John B. Murphy, M. D., at Mercy Hospital, Chicago Cal State J Med. 1912 May; 10(5): 216-217.
- O'Conner, JL, Bloom DA, William T. Bovie and electrosurgery. Surgery. 1996 Apr;119(4):390-6.
- Bovie, WT; Cushing, H (1928). "Electrosurgery as an aid to the removal of intracranial tumors with a preliminary note on a new surgical-current generator". *Surg Gynecol Obstet* **47**: 751-84.
- Heaton, LD; Ravdin, IS; Blades, B; Whelan, TJ. President Eisenhower's operation for regional enteritis: a footnote to history. *Annals of Surgery.* 1964; 159:661-666. [a] p. 664

Electronic Media

- Wikipedia contributors, "Hippocrates," *Wikipedia, The Free Encyclopedia,* http://en.wikipedia.org/w/index.php?title=Hippocrates&oldid=511287983
- Wikipedia contributors, "Barber's pole," *Wikipedia, The Free Encyclopedia,* http://en.wikipedia.org/w/index.php?title=Barber%27s_pole&oldid=508783786

- Wikipedia contributors, "Rod of Asclepius," Wikipedia, The Free Encyclopedia, http://en.wikipedia.org/w/index. php?title=Rod_of_Asclepius&oldid=513938368
- Wikipedia contributors, "Achilles' heel," *Wikipedia, The Free Encyclopedia,* http://en.wikipedia.org/w/index.php? title=Achilles%27_heel&oldid=511921150
- Wikipedia contributors, "Saints Cosmas and Damian," *Wikipedia, The FreeEncyclopedia,* http://en.wikipedia.org/ w/index.php?title=Saints_Cosmas_and_Damian&oldid= 511156578
- Wikipedia contributors, "Caesarean section," *Wikipedia, The Free Encyclopedia,* http://en.wikipedia.org/w/index. php?title=Caesarean_section&oldid=511212080
- Caesarean Section—A Brief History. U.S. National library of Medicine. National Institutes of Health. http://www.nlm.nih. gov/exhibition/cesarean/index.html
- Wikipedia contributors, "Andreas Vesalius," *Wikipedia, The Free Encyclopedia,* http://en.wikipedia.org/w/index.php?title= Andreas_Vesalius&oldid=509637522
- Wikipedia contributors, "William Harvey," *Wikipedia, The Free Encyclopedia,* http://en.wikipedia.org/w/index.php?title= William_Harvey&oldid=514341583
- Wikipedia contributors, "Anesthesia," *Wikipedia, The Free Encyclopedia,* http://en.wikipedia.org/w/index.php?title=An esthesia&oldid=508841939
- Wikipedia contributors, "Crawford Long," *Wikipedia, The Free Encyclopedia,* http://en.wikipedia.org/w/index.php? title=Crawford_Long&oldid=505221569
- Wikipedia contributors, "History of general anesthesia," *Wikipedia, The Free Encyclopedia* http://en.wikipedia. org/w/index.php?title=History_of_general_anesthesia &oldid=504700276
- Wikipedia contributors, "Ignaz Semmelweis," *Wikipedia, The Free Encyclopedia,* http://en.wikipedia.org/w/index. php?title=Ignaz_Semmelweis&oldid=518740919

- Wikipedia contributors, "Spontaneous generation," *Wikipedia, The Free Encyclopedia,* http://en.wikipedia.org/w/index.php?title=Spontaneous_generation&oldid=509802350
- Wikipedia contributors, "Joseph Lister, 1st Baron Lister," *Wikipedia, The Free Encyclopedia,* http://en.wikipedia.org/w/index.php?title=Joseph_Lister,_1st_Baron_Lister&oldid=512950238
- Wikipedia contributors, "Blood transfusion," *Wikipedia, The Free Encyclopedia,* http://en.wikipedia.org/w/index.php?title=Blood_transfusion&oldid=512996964
- The American Red Cross: The History of Blood Transfusion http://www.redcrossblood.org/learn-about-blood/history-blood-transfusion
- Wikipedia contributors, 'Ephraim McDowell', *Wikipedia, The Free Encyclopedia,* 19 March 2012, 11:59 UTC, <http://en.wikipedia.org/w/index.php?title=Ephraim_McDowell&oldid=482710291
- Wikipedia contributors, "Theodor Billroth," *Wikipedia, The Free Encyclopedia,* http://en.wikipedia.org/w/index.php?title=Theodor_Billroth&oldid=503562802
- McCarty, A.C History Appendicitis Vermiformis, Its Diseases and Treatments.www.innominatesociety.com/Articles/History%20of%20Appendicitis.htm
- Wikipedia contributors, "Hugh H. Young," *Wikipedia, The Free Encyclopedia,* http://en.wikipedia.org/w/index.php?title=Hugh_H._Young&oldid=505720984
- Wikipedia contributors, "White coat," *Wikipedia, The Free Encyclopedia,* http://en.wikipedia.org/w/index.php?title=White_coat&oldid=510398835
- Wikipedia contributors, 'Scrubs (clothing)', *Wikipedia, The Free Encyclopedia,* 20 August 2012, 12:32 UTC, <http://en.wikipedia.org/w/index.php?title=Scrubs_(clothing)&oldid=508281825
- History of Surgical Technicians. http://www.dorkbotdfw.org/history-of-surgical-technicians/

- Wikipedia contributors, "Surgical technologist," *Wikipedia, The Free Encyclopedia,* http://en.wikipedia.org/w/index. php?title=Surgical_technologist&oldid=519274768
- Wolfe, K. http://ezinearticles.comThe-History-of-Surgical-Technology&id=4614714
- Wikipedia contributors, "Howard Atwood Kelly," *Wikipedia, The Free Encyclopedia,* http://en.wikipedia.org/w/index. php?title=Howard_Atwood_Kelly&oldid=515841556
- Myron Firth Metzenbaum http://www.whonamedit.com/ doctor.cfm/3550.html
- Wikipedia contributors, "William Stewart Halsted," *Wikipedia, The Free Encyclopedia,* http://en.wikipedia.org/w/index. php?title=William_Stewart_Halsted&oldid=514773565
- Wikipedia contributors, "Edoardo Bassini," *Wikipedia, The Free Encyclopedia,* http://en.wikipedia.org/w/index. php?title=Edoardo_Bassini&oldid=516941276
- Edoardo Bassini, http://www.whonamedit.com/doctor.cfm/ 3213.html
- Harvey Williams Cushing, http://www.whonamedit.com/ doctor.cfm/980.html
- Wikipedia contributors, 'Harvey Williams Cushing', *Wikipedia, The Free Encyclopedia,* 27 July 2012, 10:14 UTC, <http:// en.wikipedia.org/w/index.php?title=Harvey_Williams_ Cushing&oldid=504405268
- Harvey Cushing: a Journey Through his Life http://www. med.yale.edu/library/historical/cushing/education.html
- Wikipedia contributors, "William Ladd," *Wikipedia, The Free Encyclopedia,* http://en.wikipedia.org/w/index. php?title=William_Ladd&oldid=517102970
- Wikipedia contributors, "William E. Ladd," *Wikipedia, The Free Encyclopedia,* http://en.wikipedia.org/w/index. php?title=William_E._Ladd&oldid=506567122
- Wikipedia contributors, 'Michael E. DeBakey', *Wikipedia, The Free Encyclopedia,* 15 October 2012, 22:55 UTC, <http://en.wikipedia.org/w/index.php?title=Michael_ E._DeBakey&oldid=518015633

- http://www.biography.com/people/michael-debakey-9269009
- Wikipedia contributors, "J. Marion Sims," *Wikipedia, The Free Encyclopedia*, http://en.wikipedia.org/w/index.php?title=J._Marion_Sims&oldid=507062800
- Alfred Blalock. http://www.whonamedit.com/doctor.cfm/2036.html
- Wikipedia contributors, 'Alfred Blalock', *Wikipedia, The Free Encyclopedia*, 11 September 2012, 21:52 UTC, <http://en.wikipedia.org/w/index.php?title=Alfred_Blalock&oldid=511918274
- http://jeffline.tju.edu/SML/Archives/Highlights/Gibbon/
- Wikipedia contributors, 'John Benjamin Murphy', *Wikipedia, The Free Encyclopedia*, 6 June 2012, 05:48 UTC, <http://en.wikipedia.org/w/index.php?title=John_Benjamin_Murphy&oldid=496229287>
- http://inventors.about.com/library/inventors/blheartlungmachine.htm
- Wikipedia contributors, "Surgical technologist," *Wikipedia, The Free Encyclopedia*, http://en.wikipedia.org/w/index.php?title=Surgical_technologist&oldid=519274768
- Wikipedia contributors, 'Emil Theodor Kocher', *Wikipedia, The Free Encyclopedia*, 5 October 2012, 06:20 UTC, <http://en.wikipedia.org/w/index.php?title=Emil_Theodor_Kocher&oldid=516102025>
- http://www.nobelprize.org/nobel_prizes/medicine/laureates/1909/kocher-bio.html
- Wikipedia contributors, "Allvar Gullstrand," *Wikipedia, The Free Encyclopedia*, http://en.wikipedia.org/w/index.php?title=Allvar_Gullstrand&oldid=517146049
- http://www.nobelprize.org/nobel_prizes/medicine/laureates/1911/gullstrand-bio.html
- http://www.nobelprize.org/nobel_prizes/medicine/laureates/1912/carrel-bio.html
- http://www.nobelprize.org/nobel_prizes/medicine/laureates/1914/barany.html

- http://www.nobelprize.org/nobel_prizes/medicine/laureates/1923/
- Wikipedia contributors, "Werner Forssmann," *Wikipedia, The Free Encyclopedia,* http://en.wikipedia.org/w/index.php?title=Werner_Forssmann&oldid=507737562 http://www.nobelprize.org/nobel_prizes/medicine/laureates/1949/hess-bio.html
- http://www.nobelprize.org/nobel_prizes/medicine/laureates/1945/fleming-bio.html
- http://www.nobelprize.org/nobel_prizes/medicine/laureates/1966/huggins-lecture.html ttp://www.nobelprize.org/nobel_prizes/medicine/laureates/1990/murray-autobio.html
- www.valleylabeducation.org/esself-2a/pages/esself2-03.html
- http://www.healthmedialab.com/html/president/early.html
- http://www.healthmedialab.com/html/president/shot.html
- Wikipedia contributors, 'Alexis Carrel', *Wikipedia, The Free Encyclopedia,* 11 October 2012, 03:30 UTC, <http://en.wikipedia.org/w/index.php?title=Alexis_Carrel&oldid=517125985
- Wikipedia contributors, "Assassination of James A. Garfield," *Wikipedia, The Free Encyclopedia,* http://en.wikipedia.org/w/index.php?title=Assassination_of_James_A._Garfield&oldid=517520913
- http://www.boatus.com/magazine/2011/october/conspiracy.asp

Made in the USA
Lexington, KY
02 December 2016